WITHDRAWN

Carnegie Mellon

GARLAND STUDIES ON

THE ELDERLY
IN AMERICA

edited by
STUART BRUCHEY
UNIVERSITY OF MAINE

A GARLAND SERIES

RACIAL DIFFERENCES IN PERCEPTIONS OF ACCESS TO HEALTH CARE AMONG THE ELDERLY

SHULAMIT L. BERNARD

GARLAND PUBLISHING, Inc.
New York & London / 1997

362.19897
R52r

Copyright © 1997 Shulamit L. Bernard
All rights reserved

Library of Congress Cataloging-in-Publication Data

Bernard, Shulamit L., 1951–
    Racial differences in perceptions of access to health care
among the elderly / Shulamit L. Bernard.
        p.   cm. — (Garland studies on the elderly in America)
    Revision of the author's thesis (Ph. D.)—University of North
Carolina at Chapel Hill, 1994.
    Includes bibliographical references and index.
    ISBN 0-8153-2646-7 (alk. paper)
    1. Afro-American aged—Medical care—North Carolina.
2. Rural aged—Medical care—North Carolina. 3. Aged—Medical
care—North Carolina. 4. Medical care—Utilization—North
Carolina. 5. Health services accessibility—North Carolina—
Public opinion. 6. Aged—North Carolina—Attitudes. 7. Medical
care—North Carolina—Public opinion. 8. Discrimination in
medical care—North Carolina. I. Title. II. Series.
RA408.M54B47 1997
362.1'9897'009756—dc21
                                                        96-39994

Printed on acid-free, 250-year-life paper
Manufactured in the United States of America

CONTENTS

With Love to . . .
Stephen, Seth and Ariele.

University Libraries
Carnegie Mellon University
Pittsburgh PA 15213-3890

yil
Ceas

LIST OF TABLES

LIST OF FIGURES

ACKNOWLEDGMENTS

I would like to thank the following colleagues and mentors for their contributions to the development of this work: Susan I. DesHarnais, Gordon H. DeFriese, Gerda G. Fillenbaum, Joanne Garrett, Thomas R. Konrad, and Jean Kincade.

With gratitude I acknowledge the receipt of a Pre- and Post-Doctoral National Research Service Award from the Agency for Health Care Policy and Research, during which time I was able to take advantage of the abundant resources, both of materials and people, that the Cecil G. Sheps Center for Health Services Research, University of North Carolina at Chapel Hill, had to offer. This experience was extremely significant to the completion of this work, as well as to my development as a researcher. I am indebted to Gordon DeFriese, and to many others at the Center, for the invaluable opportunity that I was granted.

I would like to express my gratitude to Duke University and to the staff of the Piedmont Health Survey of the Elderly for the use of the baseline data. In particular, I would like to thank Richard Landerman for his assistance with imputed data, Connie Service for coordinating the data request, and Bruce Burchett for his valuable assistance with data transfer.

Thanks also to Roger Growe for his assistance with layout and formatting of the book.

I am indebted to my family, my husband, Stephen, and children, Seth and Ariele, for their love and support.

Racial Differences in Perceptions of Access to Health Care among the Elderly

I

Introduction

Since its inception in 1965, the aim of the Medicare program has been to reduce financial barriers to hospital and physician services for the elderly population in the United States. Since that time, virtually the entire population 65 years of age and over has been entitled to hospital services covered by Medicare (Part A) and entitled to enroll voluntarily in Medicare's Part B physician's and related services program. The Medicare program was expected to (and has) improve access to physicians' services for all the Nation's elderly, however, some discrepancies in access to health care services have not fully disappeared (McBean and Gornick, 1994). Substantial differences by race have been found in rates of surgical procedures (McBean, Warren and Babish, 1994), rates of cardiac catheterization procedures (Udvarhelyi et al., 1992; Whittle et al., 1993), and rates of important diagnostic procedures (Escarce et al., 1993). In all these reported findings, rates were significantly greater in white Medicare beneficiaries compared with black beneficiaries. One of the aims of this research is to examine perceptions of access to Medical Care and perceptions of efficacy of medical care by black and white elderly community residents. Further, this study examines whether these perceptions alter medical care seeking behaviors. If black elderly are found to hold negative views of the potential benefit of medical care and as a result avoid physician visits, then it may suggest one possible explanation for the apparent discrepancy in utilization rates.

OVERVIEW

The well-documented aging of America will result in tremendous growth in the proportion of the population aged 65 and older during the early part of the 21st Century. The United States elderly population increased by 22 percent during the 1980s and is projected to grow 73 percent during the first thirty years of the next century (Taeuber, 1992). This projected change in the age structure of the American population, accompanied by an increase in the proportion of aged minorities in the population, make planning and providing health care services for elderly

Americans a major challenge. Understanding utilization behaviors of elderly community residents, their perceptions of barriers to health care services, and the relationship between perceived barriers and utilization will contribute to inform health policy for an aging population.

In recent years the relationship between age and health care services utilization has been the subject of considerable research (e.g., Segall and Chappell, 1989; Wolinsky et al., 1983; Wolinsky and Johnson, 1991). With the exception of a few studies that examined failure to use services (see for example, Stoller, 1982; Branch and Nemeth, 1985), the focus of research in this area has been on determinants of utilization. Several factors heighten the relevance of understanding elderly users and non-users of health care services in the coming decades, including: 1) the projected growth in the size of the elderly population, particularly the growth in the percentage of African-American elderly who are more likely to be in poorer health and impoverished; 2) the growing fiscal concern regarding the solvency of the Medicare program resulting from increasing expenditures and emphasis on high technological intervention; and 3) the debate regarding the extent and role of morbidity in shaping old age (Fries, 1990; Olshansky et al, 1991).

Fries (1990) contends that the period of morbidity (average age at first infirmity and the average age at death) can be compressed by advances in medical interventions resulting in a reduction in the national illness burden. Alternatively, Olshansky and colleagues (1991) argue that declines in mortality will lead to worsening health and a longer duration of life spent in a state of chronic illness and disability, resulting in a rise in the illness burden and medical expenditures. While the role of medical care in this debate is not clear, quality of life can be enhanced by the prevention of complications from existing chronic illness and possibly by early detection of disease. This can be accomplished only if elderly individuals are aware of their need for services and seek medical care in a timely fashion for symptoms and/or preventive services.

Research on the health care delivery system has identified a number of factors related to use of health care services by older adults living in the community. Andersen and colleagues formulated a model that incorporates many of these factors in specified relationships (Andersen, 1968; Andersen and Newman, 1973). This framework has been used extensively in studies of physician use by elderly people (see reviews by Wan 1989; Wolinsky 1990), and has been selected as the framework for this study.

Although health care use increases with age, differential access to care for vulnerable groups of older people is a concern. Many people do not seek medical care for significant symptoms, perhaps because they consider them the inevitable consequences of aging (Branch and Nemeth, 1985; Kane and Kane, 1990) or, despite great strides made by the Medicare program, disadvantaged elderly people continue to encounter barriers to access. Although the Medicare program has been very effective in increasing access to Medical Care for elderly people, policy trajectories since the 1980s may have resulted in issues of access (for example, cost of care) re-emerging as significant barriers to the use health care for some elderly people. As a consequence of the inflation in health care costs for nearly two decades, health care is consuming an ever greater proportion of the elderly's income (Select Committee on Aging, U.S. House of Representatives, 1994). In addition, racial differences among elderly people in delaying medical care for reasons of affordability or acceptability of care have not been clearly delineated.

This work uses Andersen's multivariable model of health service use to examine racial differences in perceptions of access to Medical Care by elderly community residents and variation in physician use resulting from these perceptions. This book includes an exploration of the role of race as mediating the decision to seek medical care. In addition, the analysis discussed here accounts for perceptions of access and attitudes toward medical care. This work therefore responds to many criticisms of prior research using the health behavior model of health service use among elderly people.

SPECIFIC AIMS OF THE STUDY

Using secondary data, this study addresses the extent to which issues of *perceived* access and/or attitudinal barriers alter the use of physician visits among elderly community residents. Both contact and volume of physician services are explored examining both direct and indirect effects of predisposing, enabling and need-for-care characteristics of the individual. While other researchers have used the health behavior model to assess the determinants of medical care utilization among elderly people, the analyses presented in this book examine the role of perceived deterrents to seeking medical care. In this way, the decision *not* to seek medical care in the presence of need is emphasized. The work contributes to our insight into why older adults decide to use, or not use, the health care system as well as to our knowledge about racial differences in perceptions of access and utilization. The research reported here addresses the following questions:

Who delays seeking medical care when there is a need to go, and why?

Does the pattern of physician visits differ for elders who delay medical care because of access concerns (i.e., financial, distance or transportation), versus elders who delay medical care because of attitudinal reasons?

Does race mediate delay in seeking medical care or use of physician visits?

The first question examines the characteristics associated with delay, and whether, in a well insured elderly population, delay in seeking medical care is attributed to issues of access or to attitudinal barriers. Question two explores whether perceptions of access or efficacy alter the likelihood of entry into the health care system and/or extent of service use. Finally, the third question investigates the role of race in the decision to delay medical care: do elderly blacks and elderly whites report similar rates of delay; do they delay for the same reasons; does delay have similar implications for physician use among the two groups of elders? It is argued here that although need is the most salient determinant of use of medical care, one could perceive a need for care and then fail to initiate a physician visit because of perceptions of access to or efficacy of medical care.

While the specific aims of this work are to answer the questions posed above, the general interest is to gain a better understanding of the impact of barriers to Medical Care on the use of physician services by elderly community residents and possible explanations for variation in use by elderly blacks and elderly whites. Although others have studied use of medical care by the elderly, this book reports on perceived deterrents to use and consistency of correlates of use and non-use among African-Americans and whites.

This work contributes to our understanding of factors important in explaining the likelihood of failing to seek medical attention in the presence of need for care. By using multivariable analysis, this research identifies factors important in explaining and predicting elderly community residents at greatest risk of failing to enter the medical care system in the presence of need for care.

The book begins with a discussion of the use of health care services by elderly community residents. Theoretical and empirical literature related to the study of health care utilization related to the proposed study is then reviewed. Following a description of the conceptual model and statement of the hypotheses to be tested in Chapter III, the research design and methodology are presented in Chapter IV. Discussion of the findings is presented in Chapters V and VI.

II

Empirical Findings on the Use of Medical Care By Older Adults

USE OF HEALTH CARE SERVICES BY OLDER AMERICANS

People over the age of 65 average more physician visits, are hospitalized more often and use twice as many prescription drugs as the under age 65 population (National Center for Health Statistics, 1990). They comprise nearly 13 percent of the United States population (U.S. Bureau of the Census, 1993), but account for over one-third of the country's total health care expenditure (Waldo et al., 1989). The impression given by these statistics is of a homogeneous group of elderly people who are high users of health care services. However, thorough examination of utilization statistics reveals that the over 65 population is heterogeneous and diverse with respect to physician and hospital use. A substantial portion of the utilization attributed to them results from extensive demand generated by a relatively small subgroup (Roos and Shapiro, 1981; Mossey, Havens and Wolinsky, 1989). In 1993, about 10 percent (3.7 million) of all Medicare enrollees accounted for 70 percent ($90.2 billion) of all Medicare payments (High Cost Users of Medicare Services, 1995). This distribution of payments has remained stable during the past two decades (Kovar, 1986).

In their extensive review of major studies exploring consistency of formal health service utilization by elderly people Mossey, Havens and Wolinsky (1989) addressed two relevant questions: whether some older individuals are consistently low users of health services year after year; and, what characteristics differentiate consistently high from consistently low users, or for that matter, from inconsistent users. They found that: 1) most older individuals are consistent from year to year in their use of physician care, patterns are established and high users remain high users and low users remain low users over time; 2) a small proportion of older individuals consistently make extensive use of physician service; and 3) need, as defined by health status, is the most salient determinant of whether the individual is a consistently high, medium, or low user. These findings are in keeping with other research which has shown that variation in use of medical care among elders is largely attributed to need (Coulton and Frost, 1982).

Health status consistently predicts use of health care services with decreasing health status associated with increasing use (Counte and Glendon, 1991). However, health status, or need for care, hardly explains all the variation in health care use (McBean and Gornick, 1994). Factors, other than need, that influence older individuals' decision to seek and use health care services must be understood (Stoller and Forster, 1994).

RACIAL DIFFERENCES IN ACCESS TO AND UTILIZATION OF HEALTH CARE SERVICE

The American elderly population is becoming a more racially and ethnically diverse group. In 1990, the ratio of elderly non-whites to elderly whites was 1 in 10. Projections estimate that by the middle of the next century the ratio of black elderly to white elderly will rise to 2 in 10 (Taeuber, 1992). By the year 2,000, there will be nearly three million blacks aged 65 and over. In addition, by the year 2030 the black elderly population will more than double reaching 7.3 million persons (Parks, 1988). Blacks constitute the most rapidly growing portion of the oldest-old population (Gibson and Jackson, 1992). Overall, the number of elderly African-Americans is increasing at a rate substantially faster than that of the general population, and also at a faster rate than that of elderly whites.

Black elderly generally score lower than elderly whites on self-ratings of health status (National Center for Health Statistics, 1990), and have a shorter life expectancy than whites. Differences in life expectancy between black and whites who reach the age of 65 is increasing (Manton, Patrick and Johnson, 1987). Elderly blacks have higher rates of morbidity and mortality due to chronic illness such as ischemic heart disease (Ell et al., 1994). Findings suggest that they receive less specialized care for these conditions (McBean and Gornick, 1994). Long delay times between onset of symptoms and arrival at a hospital have been documented in this population (Cooper et al., 1986) and sociodemographic status is thought to be a factor (Jackson, 1988; James, 1989). These delays are significant because they can diminish the effectiveness of new therapies that must be given promptly at the onset of symptoms (Strogatz, 1990). Ell and colleagues (1994) examined whether African-American patients who seek prompt care have different characteristics from those who do not.

Their findings suggest that differences in care seeking behaviors in this population were found to be related to socioeconomic status.

Substantial racial differences were found in the use of medical services by elderly Americans (Escarce et al., 1993; McBean and Gornick, 1994). Using 1986 physician claims data for a national sample of Medicare enrollees Escarce and colleagues (1993) found that black elderly were less likely than white elderly to receive medical services, that race may exacerbate the impact of other barriers to access and that racial differences in use of medical services persisted even when comparisons were made among elders of similar socio-economic background (i.e., Medicaid recipients). In addition, racial differences in use are greater among elderly persons who reside in Southern rural areas. Race seems to magnify the impact of other barriers to medical care. The apparent modifying effect of race on the relationship between access and use of health care services needs to be better understood.

White elderly are more likely to purchase private insurance policies that supplement Medicare benefits as compared with black elderly (Rice and McCall, 1985). While those with supplementary insurance have been shown to use more medical care (Escarce et al., 1993; Seccombe, 1995), racial differences in purchasing supplementary insurance and subsequent perceptions regarding access and use of medical services remain to be explored.

Drawing on data from two national surveys of black Americans, the National Survey of Black Americans (NSBA) and the Three Generation Black Family Study (TGBFS) Gibson and Jackson (1992) summarize and describe the health and function of elderly black Americans. While the association between age and number of chronic conditions, age and overall health status, and age and functional status are linear among white elderly, their analysis of the data suggests that these relationships are nonlinear among blacks. However, they caution that racial disparities in health vary "according to data source and specific measure of health (p. 329)." Apparently, blacks report their health and functioning more accurately in global-subjective measures, such as self-reported health status, than in measures requiring specific recall of particular symptoms (Gibson and Jackson, 1992).

Black elderly are more likely to live in families with limited economic resources. According to the United States Bureau of the Census (1987), blacks aged 65 and over are nearly three times as likely as their white counterparts to live in families with incomes less than $5,000. They are also more likely to be in poor physical and functional health (Gibson and

Jackson, 1992). Research has begun to focus on elderly blacks, particularly those living in rural areas (Parks, 1988) in order to obtain needed descriptive data about their use of health care services. Research on the use of medical care services by black elderly as compared with white elderly provides contradictory results. The Medicare health insurance program is available to nearly all elderly Americans regardless of race or income. Despite some gaps in coverage, Medicare insurance has improved access to Medical Care among previously underserved populations (McBean and Gornick, 1994). Whereas 25 years ago, black or poor elders had considerably lower rates of physician and hospital admissions compared with their white or higher-income counterparts (Salber et al., 1973), some studies have found that the frequency of physician visits among elderly persons currently varies little by race or income (Long and Settle, 1984; Davis et al., 1987). Wolinsky (1990) found that black elderly use more health care services as compared with white elderly and attributes these differences to differences in morbidity. Findings of differential rates of utilization for black and white elderly suggest that the impact of increasing government role in third party payments for health care via Medicare and Medicaid may have been much greater for the low-income group as a whole than it has been for the white group (Andersen and Aday, 1978) and by inference, change in government policy regarding out of pocket expenses may disproportionately affect this group's ability to access care.

Contrary to the studies cited above, pervasive racial differences in the use of medical services by elderly Americans that could not be explained by differences in the prevalence of specific medical conditions have recently been reported (Escarce et al., 1993; McBean and Gornick, 1994). Findings suggest that race modifies the relationship between access barriers and utilization of medical services. Minority status impacts on health status, as indicated by differences in life expectancy between black and white elderly and differences in death rates from various causes (Manuel and Reid, 1982). Since black elderly have been shown to be less healthy than their white counterparts it can be assumed that they should use relatively more services. However, the data do not consistently support this assumption (Escarce et al., 1993; Javitt et al, 1991; McBean and Gornick, 1994). Despite a higher incidence of heart disease and cardiac arrest among blacks compared with whites, blacks are less likely to survive cardiac arrest (Becker et al., 1993) and less likely to undergo treatment procedures such as bypass surgery or angiography (Whittle et al., 1993). There is no conclusive evidence that differences in the use of health care services between elderly blacks and elderly whites can be attributed to race or whether they can be explained by socioeconomic status. In an urban population of blacks and whites who were of similar socioeconomic status, Crawford and colleagues (1994) found few racial differences in coronary heart disease-related care patterns.

Jackson and colleagues (1982) argue that elderly blacks face "double jeopardy." This hypothesis proposes that the situation of older blacks is best characterized as one resulting from the combined effects of age and race. Consequently, while both black and white aged may be handicapped by their age, black aged are also handicapped by their race. Jackson and colleagues' hypothesis does not propose that all aged blacks are equally at risk or are more disadvantaged than all aged whites, rather it suggests the existence of a "comparative average disadvantage of the black aged."

Generally, in studies of medical care utilization by elderly persons, subjects who are black or belong to another minority are grouped into one category designated as 'nonwhite'. With a few exceptions (for example, Wright, Creecy and Berg, 1979; Mutran and Ferraro, 1988; Keith and Jones, 1990), multivariate analyses rarely test for interaction between race and other explanatory variables. Consequently, questions of whether blacks and other minorities use health services for the same reasons as whites or whether variables have the same significance for minorities have not been given sufficient attention (Keith and Jones, 1990). Compared with aged whites, black elders are more likely to experience economic hardship (Manual and Reid, 1982) and to perceive their health as being poor (Gibson and Jackson, 1992). Given these disadvantages, along with the "double jeopardy" hypothesized by Jackson and colleagues (1982), it is reasonable to assume that factors such as economic status, health insurance coverage, and perceived health status may interact with race in explaining utilization patterns. Some supporting evidence for differential determinants for blacks and whites can be found in Wan's (1982) study of elderly living in low income urban areas. Although self-reported health status was the most influential factor in explaining number of physician visits in both groups, health insurance coverage was significant for blacks but not for whites. This suggests that affordability is more of a problem for blacks than for whites (Keith and Jones, 1990). While access barriers to Medical Care, such as insurance, have to some extent been studied, *perceptions* about access and attitudes toward the health care system, which influence the decision to seek medical care, among the African-American elderly population have yet to be explored.

THEORETICAL BACKGROUND IN ACCESS TO AND UTILIZATION OF MEDICAL CARE

Initiating entry into the health care system requires that the individual recognize a need for services and seek medical care. In this section, the decision to seek care is explored, followed by discussions of delaying medical care and the concept of need for medical care. Then, models of physician utilization are presented with a focus on the theoretical model of individual determinants of access and utilization of health care initially developed by Andersen and Newman (1973), revised by Aday and Andersen (1974), and adapted by numerous researchers in the field of aging. This is followed by a discussion of empirical results from studies which examined health care use by elderly people with the Andersen model as a framework.

The Decision to Seek Medical Care

A decision to seek medical care is influenced by the individual's perception of physical illness (Berkanovic, Telesky and Reeder, 1981; Rosner, Namazi, and Wykle, 1988), the belief in the efficacy of medical intervention (Krout, 1983; Yeatts, Crow and Folts, 1992) and the ability to access care (Krout, 1983; Yeatts, Crow and Folts, 1992; Farmer, 1993). Ell and colleagues (1994) found that differences in care seeking can be attributed to socioeconomic status while Stoller and Forster (1994) found that uncertainty regarding potential seriousness, level of pain or interference, were significant predictors of physician contact.

Entry into the American health care system is initiated by the individual in response to some need, generally perceived as some disturbance in health or well being. According to Donabedian (1973, p. 59):

> Usually, it is the client who must recognize need, decide to seek care, take appropriate action to seek it, and place himself under care through adopting those behaviors that are considered appropriate for persons who are ill. In some instances the route to a physician visit is circuitous and involves the advice and intervention of family members and friends, who constitute the individual's social support network as well as the 'lay referral system'. However, service use after initial entry is influenced by need, physician practice patterns and other socio-demographic variables, for example health insurance and income.

It is necessary, therefore, to differentiate between indicators of entry into the health care system and level of use (Penchansky and Thomas, 1981).

People who are poor (Weissman et al., 1991; Branch and Nemeth, 1985), black, uninsured, with grade school education (Weissman et al., 1991), having low morale and diminished health status (Safer et al., 1979) are more likely to report instances of not going to the doctor when they think they should. Time between the decision to seek care and a physician visit is shortest for persons who are not concerned about the cost of care (Ell et al., 1994) and who are certain that symptoms could be addressed by the physician (Safer et al., 1979; Stoller and Forster, 1994).

Delaying Medical Care

Few studies have examined the correlates and implications of delaying medical care among older people (see for example, Yeatts, Crow and Folts, 1992; Branch and Nemeth, 1985). Findings among the few studies that have indicate that elderly people postpone or delay medical care for significant symptoms because they attribute them to age (Branch and Nemeth, 1985) or, particularly among elderly people living at or below poverty, concern about cost is given as a reason for delay (Stoller, 1982; Branch and Nemeth, 1985; Kane and Kane, 1990). Although people aged 65 and over average more physician visits than younger people, studies have shown that only a small proportion of elders account for a large share of the services used (Roos and Shapiro, 1981; Kovar, 1986). High utilization of medical care among elderly people has been attributed primarily to health status and need for care (see Coulton and Frost, 1982; Counte and Glandon, 1991; Kelman and Thomas, 1988; Wolinsky and Coe, 1984). However, despite the nearly universal health care coverage for Americans aged 65 and over, there remains an important component of this population who fail to seek or postpone care seeking when perceiving a need (Stoller and Forster, 1994). Phenomena, other than need for care, which significantly influence elderly persons' decision to seek medical care need to be defined, measured and addressed by health policy.

Given the high rate of chronic and debilitating diseases among the elderly, low rates of physician utilization are particularly worrisome in this population. Elderly people with chronic disease may ignore warning signs of serious conditions if they attribute them to aging (Stoller, 1982; Stoller and Forster, 1994). Even with respect to less potentially threatening conditions, lack of prompt attention to symptoms could result in unnecessary complications by hindering medical intervention for avoidable or treatable conditions (Ell et al., 1994).

Much of the emphasis in research of health care use by elderly people focuses on volume of services used and on relationships between specific indicators (e.g., health status, socio-demographic, health insurance) and type and amount of utilization. During 1989 over 80 percent of elderly people had at least one annual visit with a physician (National Center for Health Statistics, 1990). Depending on year and source of data, between 15 and 20 percent of elderly people have no contact with a physician during the course of a year (Branch and Nemeth, 1985; Shapiro and Roos, 1985; National Center for Health Statistics, 1990) thereby forfeiting an opportunity for early detection and treatment of disease or close monitoring of chronic illness.

In a study by Stoller (1982), nearly one third of elderly persons reported putting off medical attention when they felt ill or believed they had a medical problem because of being too busy (3.8 percent), preferring to wait for a regular appointment (20.8 percent), medical care being too costly (17.4 percent), thinking a doctor could not help (25.6 percent), and not wanting to bother the doctor (14.5 percent). Stoller's findings suggest that a significant minority of older persons recognize the need for medical care but fail to seek physician services because of financial or attitudinal factors.

Concern about elderly non-users of care is legitimate. Research findings suggest that poverty, social isolation, belonging to an ethnic minority and low education attainment are attributes associated with a greater likelihood of delaying needed medical care and that such behavior is associated with longer hospital stays and higher mortality (Shapiro and Roos, 1985; Weissman et al., 1991). An examination of characteristics and health outcomes of elderly non-users of health care services in the Manitoba Longitudinal Study on Aging by Shapiro and Roos (1985) indicate that non-users were at greater risk of lengthy hospitalizations and died sooner than low users. In addition, treatment delays can result in diminished effectiveness of new treatment (Ell et al., 1994).

Using data from the third wave of the Massachusetts Health Care Panel Study, Branch and Nemeth (1985) examined reasons for instances of failing to seek medical care by elderly community residents. They found that 17 percent of their sample reported instances of failing to visit a physician when perceiving a need for a visit. Failure to visit a physician was attributed to one of four reasons: believing symptoms experienced were due to age; concern with the cost of medical care; transportation difficulties; and unavailability of an appointment. Twelve of the 17 percent who failed to visit a physician did so specifically because they believed their problem was due to age. This study controlled for health status using both self-perceived health, a functional problem index, and dependency in basic activities of daily living. Poverty, low morale and diminished health status were attributes associated with a greater likelihood of reporting instances of *not* seeing a physician for reasons of transportation difficulties, cost concerns, or attributing symptoms to age. Higher income, lack of private insurance, living alone, being male, and low morale were characteristics associated with a greater likelihood of attributing failure to visit a physician on appointment difficulties. Those who attributed their health problems to age were more likely *not* to have annual contact with a physician.

There are a number of questions left unanswered by research to date: what are the determinants of failure to seek care among black elders, are they the same or do they differ from that of white elders; and, are there geographic difference in reasons for failing to seek physician visits. The Branch and Nemeth study, as well as Stoller's and Forster's (1994) work, was conducted in the Northeast leaving one to question the generalizability of their findings to other regions.

Despite the fact that black elderly are a growing component of the aged population, that their prevalence of chronic illness is high and they are more likely to perceive their health as fair or poor, little is known about their reasons for delaying medical care. This research proposes to build on the work of Stoller (1982) and Branch and Nemeth (1985), by examining perceived access and attitudinal barriers to Medical Care comparing white and black elderly community residents.

Need for Medical Care

The concept of need for medical care is central to a discussion of medical care utilization. Need in this context has been succinctly defined by Donabedian as "some disturbance in health and well being" (1973; p. 62). Donabedian contends there is a minimum of two perspectives of need: that of the individual seeking care and that of the physician. The individual's perception determines initial contact with the health care system while both individual and physician perspectives influence volume of services.

Physician definition of need derives from training and socialization of the physician and technological offerings in the way of diagnosis and treatment, while individual perception of need reflects concern with the perceived impact of illness and interference with activities of daily living (as defined by the individual). These two perspectives result in need defined as two different dimensions which may be only partly congruent. There is a tendency in medical care planning to accept physicians' estimate of need as the more definitive one (Donabedian, 1973), often resulting in a view of the individual as making too much demand on the health care system or under utilizing medical care.

Need can also be defined in broader terms than health status. Situations in which prevention or health promotion activities are beneficial must also be included in the definition of need (for example, screening mammography). Consequently, if by virtue of age annual contact with a physician is deemed appropriate for the purposes of monitoring and screening then, in the presence of good health status and in the absence of chronic illness, there exists a 'need' for contact with a physician.

Need has consistently been shown to be the primary factor in determining use of health care among older adults. In their extensive review of studies examining utilization of medical care, Hulka and Wheat (1985) conclude that measures of need rank as the first and most important contributors to explained variance in utilization. Additionally, studies that used severity of illness condition as a proxy for dose, found evidence for a "dose-response relationship between need and utilization" (p. 441).

Because need-for-care explains a large proportion of the variation in utilization of medical care, studies that attempt to understand determinants of utilization other than need must carefully measure and control for need in analyses. Currently, there is no consistent method of defining or conceptualizing need measures. In general, need is defined and measured in two broad categories: individually perceived and professionally assessed health status (Hulka and Wheat, 1985).

MODELS OF PHYSICIAN UTILIZATION

Research has shown that use of health care services is determined by individuals' responses to their health and illness levels, as well as preconditioned by demographic, social structural, psychological, familial and community resources and health care organizational factors (Wan, 1989).

In the general population, these correlates have been studied for well over 20 years. In the past 15 years or so there has been an increased focus in the study of health care utilization among aged populations, including analyses of data gathered from both community and national health surveys (see Arling, 1985; Branch et al, 1981; Evashwich et al. 1984; Wolinsky, 1990).

In an overview of determinants of health services use among the elderly, Wan (1989) summarizes three conceptual approaches which have been used to explain the relationship between various predictors and utilization of health care services (p. 53-54):

Rosenstock's health belief model incorporates both psychological and social variables to predict utilization behavior. According to this model "readiness to seek medical care is determined by perceived susceptibility and severity of a health problem, perceived benefits and barriers to seeking care, and cues that instigate appropriate behavior" (p. 53). Analytic models developed from this approach have been applied to the general population but rarely to the elderly (see Becker and Maiman, 1983; Jette et al, 1981; or Bausell, 1986).

The second approach is the behavioral model, developed by Andersen (1968) and Andersen and Newman (1973). This framework assumes that individual variation in the use of health care services is a function of three dimensions of variables which are defined as: a) predisposing or personal attributes which predispose individuals to seek medical care; b) enabling factors such as income, insurance, and availability of a regular source of medical care which either present barriers to care by their lack of availability or enable the individual to seek care by their availability; and, 3) need for care factors including subjective, or self-perceived health and objective health status and functional level.

Wan identifies the third conceptual approach as the economic approach. The economic framework considers that variation in use of health care services is "contingent upon organizational constraints, indicated by the level of market competition and incentives for developing cost-effective alternatives for care, and personal choice or decision factors" (p. 54). The focus of this perspective is on relevant organizational or personal choice factors which facilitate or impede care seeking behaviors.

The two models which are used most frequently in empirical research will be discussed below: the health belief model, developed by Rosenstock (1974) and Andersen's (1968) model of health care utilization.

The Health Belief Model

According to the health belief model, the decision to seek medical care is contingent upon four key beliefs which must be present prior to the initiation of a physician visit (Kasl, 1974): 1) health motivation, or the belief that one is susceptible to illness; 2) belief that symptoms experienced are sufficiently severe to warrant a visit; 3) belief in the efficacy of medical intervention; and 4) belief that the cost of medical care or barriers encountered are reasonable given the need. In an attempt to integrate the role of social support in the process of seeking medical care several modifications were included (Krause, 1990). Kasl (1974) argued that members of ones social support network influence illness behavior by: 1) assisting in the interpretation of severity of symptoms; 2) suggesting actions to alleviate symptoms; and 3) providing instrumental assistance, such as transportation, to facilitate care seeking decisions. Additionally, Kirscht (1974) suggested further modifications of the model by including characteristics such as age, sex, socioeconomic status, and psychological characteristics such as alienation, fatalism and skepticism.

Although the health belief model has been discussed for nearly two decades it has not been applied extensively in empirical research. While several studies attempted to evaluate this complex model (Becker and Maiman, 1983) no attempts have been made to apply this model to the study of health care utilization among the elderly (Krause, 1990).

The Health Behavior Model

The use of medical care by older people "results from a complex set of factors involving health status, social, and psychological characteristics, and economic and organizational variables" (Arling, 1985). Andersen and colleagues (Aday and Andersen, 1975; Aday, Andersen and Fleming, 1980; Andersen and Aday, 1978) formulated a model including a wide range of variables which act as determinants of utilization. While not in the strict sense a theory, it is a "descriptive typology for relating variables which may account for the use of health care services" (Arling, 1985). This model attempts to explain variations in health service as resulting from the interplay between predisposing, enabling, and need for care factors.

According to the behavioral model some individuals have a higher propensity to use a greater number or range of health services than do others. This propensity results from certain characteristics of the individual which existed prior to the onset of a specific illness episode and comprised of predisposing factors such as age, gender, race, education and household composition.

Given that individuals have differing propensities to use health care services, some means for acquiring these services must be present which enable the individual to seek medical care. This component is called 'enabling' and it is defined by factors which make health care services more or less accessible to the individual. The enabling component is composed of two dimensions: individual and community resources. The individual resource dimension includes income, availability of health insurance, and having a regular source of care. Modifications of this model resulted in the inclusion of a measure of social support which can influence physician utilization by facilitating entry (providing transportation or concurring that a visit is appropriate). The community resource dimension includes: physician and hospital bed to population ratios, geographical location and population density of residence.

Finally, assuming that both the predisposing and enabling factors are present, the individual must recognize the presence of a specific need before initiating a physician visit. With the exception of a general measure of self-perceived health, this factor is rarely measured or included in an empirical model as the individual's perception of his or her symptoms and clinical assessment of health status. More often, measures of health status include anything from number of days spent in bed to difficulties with activities of daily living.

The last component of the model is the outcome of interest which is typically use of health care services. Andersen (1968) identified two types of use — discretionary and non-discretionary. Discretionary represents health care services whose use is driven by choice, for example, going to see the dentist. Non-discretionary represents health services whose use is decided upon by the provider, for example hospitalization. Physician use falls somewhere in the middle because the decision to initiate a visit is discretionary but physician recommendations are major determinants of frequency of follow-up visits.

REVIEW OF EMPIRICAL LITERATURE ON THE APPLICATION OF THE ANDERSEN MODEL TO THE STUDY OF THE USE OF PHYSICIAN SERVICES BY THE ELDERLY

In recent years many researchers examining physician use among elderly people have adopted and adapted the Andersen behavioral model as a framework for grouping determinants of physician utilization. This model has been applied in the analysis of survey data, much of which has been large and representative of the older population. Wolinsky (1990) identifies four reasons why the behavioral model has become and remains quite popular in studies of health care utilization: 1) it is eclectic in approach, combining a "diversity of discipline-oriented perspectives"; 2) it permits an assessment of the equity in the distribution health services utilization that has considerable importance for policy makers; 3) unlike the health belief model, it can be easily applied to survey data; and 4) the behavioral model has considerable "intuitive appeal". Despite this appeal, results have "cast doubt on the power or general utility of the model in explaining health services use" (Arling, 1985). Application of the model to older people has explained only between 10 and 25 percent of the variance in the use of health care services, and need variables have accounted for most of this variance (see for example, Branch et al., 1981; Coulton and Frost, 1982; Wan, 1982; Wolinsky and Coe, 1984). This reflects less explained variance in this groups' health services utilization than for the general United States population (Wan, 1989). While some researchers suggest that the importance of predisposing and enabling characteristics have been eroded by programs (such as Medicare) targeted for older Americans (see Bice, Eichhorn and Fox, 1972; Wolinsky, 1981; Haug, 1981), alternative explanation have been offered (see Wolinsky et al., 1983; Wolinsky and Coe 1984; Arling, 1985). These include: a) imprecise measurements of health beliefs and health status; and, b) failure to account for the interaction between health, functional impairment, and economic status.

Many studies have employed multivariate analysis techniques, such as path analysis and regression, to explore the relative importance of predisposing, enabling and need-for-care characteristics in explaining the variance in number of physician visits or probability of an annual visit. A listing of selected studies relevant to this discussion are summarized in Table 2.1, with a brief summary of each study given below. These studies illustrate the evolution in the application of the Andersen model by successive researchers in the field of aging in an attempt to better understand health and illness behavior of older adults.

Table 2.1: Empirical studies of health care use with Andersen's health behavior model as the conceptual framework.

Author (s)	Sample	Need Variables	Predisposing Variables	Enabling Variables	Physician Visits
Wright, Creecy and Berg (1979)	Community health survey of black low-income elderly residing in public housing in Milwaukee, WI N = 414	Self Reported Health* Number of Health Conditions Number of Disability Days*	Age Sex Marital Status Morale * Education	Income Health Insurance Regular Source of Care *	Number of Physician Visits during previous 12 months
Branch et al. (1981)	Massachusetts - statewide area probability sample N = 1,625	Self -Perceived health status* Katz ADL scale Rosow-Breslow: perform physical exercise* climb stairs* walk 1/2 mile Health Problems	Age Gender Race Education Household Composition Marital Status	Income Occupational Status Medicaid Coverage VA Coverage Private Health Insurance Regular Physician* Transportation Problems	Number of physician contacts
Coulton and Frost (1982)	Study of Older People in Cleveland Ohio 1975-76 N = 1,834	Mental Impairment* ADL and IADL Perceived need for service*	Sex Race Social Isolation* Subjective psychological distress	Income Health Insurance: no benefits hospital benefits only hospital and ambulatory Education Case Management*	Frequency of physician visits

* indicate variables found to be statistically significant at p<.05.

Author (s)	Sample	Need Variables	Predisposing Variables	Enabling Variables	Physician Visits
Stoller (1982)	Non-institutionalized older persons living in a 17 county region of Northeastern New York (N = 753)	Worry about health * (volume) # symptoms Ill in bed during previous year * (contact) Health interferes with desired activities * (volume) Physician evaluation of need * (contact and volume)	Age * (volume) Sex * (contact) Marital Status Household composition * (volume) Education * (contact) Health attitudes Rural * (volume)	Health Insurance: Medicare part A Medicare A and B * (volume) Medicaid * (volume) Physician/pop. ratio for county * (contact) Convenience to doctor * (contact and volume) Usual source: local doctor, emergency room or out patient department * (volume)	Physician Contact (yes/no) Volume among users of care
Wolinsky et al. (1983)	Elderly residents of south central metropolitan St. Louis (N = 401)	Perceived health* Mental orientation Katz functional status Instrumental ADL Sensory function Nutritional risk* Morale scale	Age Sex Marital Status Living alone Race (black/white) Locus of Control Nutritional Knowledge	Income Health Insurance Regular Physician *	Preventive medicine contacts Total doctor visits Total emergency room visits Hospitalization

24

Author (s)	Sample	Need Variables	Predisposing Variables	Enabling Variables	Physician Visits
Evashwick et al., (1984)	Massachusetts Health Care Panel Study N = 1,317	Modified Katz ADL Scale Modified Rosow-Breslow scale* Self-Reported Health Status* Self-Reported Physical Conditions*	Age Sex Race (white/other) Education Living Alone Married Widowed Seeing a physician on a regular basis*	Occupation Income Insurance: Medicaid* VA insurance private insurance Have own doctor* No transportation problems*	Any Physician services during 15 months preceding the interview (yes/no)
Wolinsky and Coe (1984)	1978 Health Interview Survey (sample aged 60 and over) N = 15,899	Limited activity* Overall health* Body mass ratio	Sex* Age Married* Widowed* Lives Alone* Race (white/nonwhite)* Education Employed*	Regular source of care* Telephone* Income* Health insurance: Private* Medicaid* Medicare* Region* Rural/urban*	Physician visits truncated at 13 or more

25

Author (s)	Sample	Need Variables	Predisposing Variables	Enabling Variables	Physician Visits
Arling (1985)	1979 Survey of Older Virginians N= 2,146	Medical Conditions* ADL -Impairment	Age* Race - (white/other) Sex Education* Marital Status Living Alone	Poverty* Social Support* Source of Medical Care Insurance Coverage Psychosomatic Distress Scale* Emotional Distress Scale*	Number of visits - ranging from (-20 during the 6 months preceding the interview.
Mutran and Ferraro (1988)	1973 Survey of the Low Income Aged andDisabled (SLIAD): the Current Population Survey of Low Income Subsample was used. (N = 3,150)	Chronic Illness Serious Illness * Disability * Self-Assessed Health*	Gender Race (white/other) Education * Age	Income * Urban Residence Proximity to Children* Marital Status Medicaid Enrollment*	Physician Visits during the past year (yes/no)

Author (s)	Sample	Need Variables	Predisposing Variables	Enabling Variables	Physician Visits
Eve (1988)	Social Security Administration's Longitudinal Retirement History Survey - subsample of older women without a spouse N = 3,013	Handicapped or disabled* Subjective Health*	Age Widowed Divorced Never Married Education Race (white/other) Head of Household Living children* Retired Previous health status	Annual Family Income Satisfaction with income Ability to get along with income Health Insurance* Previous use of health care*	Physician visits during previous year ranging 0 - 21 (truncated at 21); Put off care during previous year
Keith and Jones (1990)	1975 National Survey of the Aged N = 1,902 (1,505 whites and 397 blacks)	Morale Loneliness Health Status* (whites and blacks) Index of Incapacity	Age Sex* (whites only) Education* (whites only) Widowed* (blacks only) Living Alone (both whites and blacks) In labor force (blacks only)	Income Place of residence (farm to metro)* (blacks only) Private Health Insurance* (whites only)	Physician Contact (yes/no)

* statistically significant at p>.05

In making comparisons across studies it should be noted that although all of these studies use Andersen's health behavior model as a framework, the precise specification of the empirical model varies from study to study. In one of the only studies that specifically applies the Andersen model to a black elderly population Wright, Creecy and Berg (1979), examine a causal model of health care use by low-income black elderly residing in public housing projects in Milwaukee. Their findings indicate that four of the explanatory variables (number of reported illness conditions, existence of a regular source of medical care, self-perceived health status and morale or life satisfaction) have a direct effect on physician utilization and, in combination account for 26 percent of the explained variance. Socio-demographic variables such as age, education and income have an indirect effect on physician utilization through their relationship with self-perceived health status. This work marks an important beginning in the understanding of utilization of services among elderly blacks, however, there are several limitations to the study. These include: 1) a sample limited to low income urban black elderly; 2) no differentiation between predictors of contact and volume of services; 3) lack of social support measures other than marital status; and 4) poor operationalization of the health insurance measure.

Using data from a 1974 Massachusetts statewide survey Branch and colleagues (1981), found that need for care factors (defined as poor health, limited physical activity and chronic conditions) were positively associated with use of physician services among elderly community residents. As with the Wright, Creecy and Berg (1979) study, the only predisposing or enabling variable found to be a significant predictor of physician utilization was the availability of a regular source of care. In this study health insurance is well defined and included in the empirical model as a series of dummy variables such as Medicare, Medicaid, Veterans Administration (VA) and private. However, the study does not differentiate contact from volume and although race is included in the analysis whites comprised 99 percent of the sample.

In a study of health care utilization by elderly people living in Cleveland, Ohio, Coulton and Frost (1982) included a measure of social isolation and psychological distress. Socially isolated elders were found to be more inclined to be low users of medical care; this finding has implications for the role of social support in the utilization of health care services. This study also included both physical and cognitive impairment as need-for-care factors to determine which aspect of impairment is associated with variation in use of physician services. Once need was accounted for in the multivariate analysis, enabling and predisposing factors contributed little to the explained variance. The major contribution of this work lies in its introduction of social isolation and psychological distress to the behavioral model and the application of the model to use of community services as well as physician care. However, the study does not differentiate between contact and volume of services and does not adequately explore the relevance of this model for black elderly.

Using a probability sample of 753 older persons living in a 17 county region of northeastern New York, Stoller (1982) applied hierarchical multiple regression techniques to assess the impact of objective and subjective need, financial resources availability and accessibility of services, attitudes toward health and medical care, and social structural and demographic characteristics on *both* physician contact and volume of services. A major contribution of this paper lies in defining the outcome variable, use of physician services, in terms of both contact and volume resulting in the finding that predictors of contact with a physician differ from predictors of volume of services. While need was found to be the major determinant of volume of services among users of care, attitudinal and background characteristics were more important in explaining initial contact. Among enabling factors, availability and accessibility of services were relatively more important in predicting initial contact while financial resources were the most important predictors of volume. This study suggests that different factors are involved in predicting contact with a physician and volume of physician visits. Need factors make a greater contribution in explaining the volume of visits than in predicting initial contact. Among the need variables, the number of clinically significant symptoms reported by the older person was the best predictor of initial contact with a physician while more subjective measures of health were found to be the best predictors of the number of visits. Enabling factors such as insurance coverage of physician visits and having a regular source of care were found to be significant in predicting volume but not initial contact.

Data from a sample of 401 elderly residents of south central St. Louis were used by Wolinsky and colleagues (1983) to assess health services utilization among the non-institutionalized elderly. Using an extensive set of measures for predisposing, enabling and need for care factors they defined the outcome related to physician use in two ways: whether the individual had a preventive medical contact with a physician and total doctor visits. They included health status indicators measures such as nutritional risk, sensory function and morale scale. A total of seven need-for-care measures were included but none noted the presence of chronic conditions or of diagnosed illness. The findings supported Stoller's (1982) work; different factors were found to be involved with the probability of having a preventive medical contact and total doctor visits. For example, as self-perceived health status improved the number of physician visits decreased, however, this measure had no influence on the probability of a preventive medical contact. In addition, while sensory function was associated with an increase in the probability of having a preventive medical contact it had no influence on the number of physician visits. Having a regular source of care was positively related to both outcomes. Although two outcome measures were used for physician care, the number of physician visits ranged from zero to twelve visits. This definition differs from Stoller (1982) who examined predictors of volume of visits among *users* of care.

Evashwick and colleagues (1984), used data from a needs assessment, conducted by the Massachusetts Department of Public Health, of 1,317 people over the age of 65 who participated in a 1974 interview and 1976 follow-up. The purpose of their research was to identify factors explaining utilization of both health and social services by older people. They evaluated the effect of predisposing, enabling and need for care factors on utilization, one factor at a time and simultaneously. Although predisposing and enabling variables were found to be of minor predictive value compared with need variables, their findings indicate that the model should include all three concepts and caution must be used in assessing the impact of one of the three constructs independently of the others. In other words, although predisposing and enabling factors were not strongly associated with physician visits they confound the relationship between need-for-care and utilization and therefore, must be included in the model. This study however, does not differentiate contact with a physician and volume of services and, the sample included too few black elderly to evaluate the effect of race on utilization.

The studies reviewed thus far relied on regional data to assess the effects of Andersen's health behavior model on utilization of health care services by older adults. In 1984, Wolinsky and Coe reported on an analysis of the 1978 Health Interview Survey which included data on 15,899 noninstitutionalized elderly people. One of the purposes of the study was to determine "if the parameters of Andersen's model estimated in these national data differed substantially from those estimated in prior regional applications of the model" (p. 334). They used multiple regression analysis and coded the outcome variable in three ways: 1) the actual number of visits to physicians during the preceding 12 month period, 2) a recoding of the actual number of physician visits that truncated the distribution so that 13 or more visits were considered as 13 visits, and 3) the natural logarithm of the actual number of physician visits. In this way they were able to address two issues related to the poor predictive ability of the Andersen model: a) whether this has been an issue of regional versus national data, and/or, b) whether this has been a function of failure to adjust for the non-normally distributed health services utilization measure. Wolinsky and Coe (1984) found no evidence that the predictability of this model is systematically affected in regional data sets. However, the data showed significant increases in the predictive utility of the behavioral model when physician visits was truncated or transformed logarithmically. For example, when the actual number of physician visits was used as the outcome variable, the model (which included predisposing, enabling and need-for-care characteristics) explained 3.9 percent of the variance in utilization; when the truncated measure was used 20 percent of the variance was explained and when the logged version was used 21.3 percent of the variance was explained. In addition, the significance of individual regression coefficients varied depending on the coding of the outcome variable. Taken together, these findings support the need for adjusting statistical methods before concluding that the conceptual framework of the model needs adjustment. Wolinsky and Coe (1984) concluded that the behavioral model is "an appropriate one for use with modest to moderate users of health services. The behavioral model, however, appears not to be appropriate for heavy users of health services" (p.341).

Arling (1985) argued that previous studies using multivariable models of physician visits by older people failed to take into account the interaction between health, functional impairment, and economic status. Analyzing data from a Virginia statewide survey of 2,146 noninstitutionalized older people he found that: a) low income had a negative main effect and a negative interaction effect (with medical conditions) on the number of physician visits; b) the number and self-perceived severity of medical conditions were important predictors of the number of physician visits for those *without* functional impairment but these factors were not significant among functionally impaired individuals; and c) social support was a major factor accounting for visits among the functionally impaired. While the interaction terms introduced in the model did not explain a great deal of additional variance they did reveal effects of theoretical importance. These findings indicate that the effects of 'need' on physician visits are not uniform and both main and interaction effects must be considered in analysis for improved understanding of the underlying process (Ronis and Harrison, 1988).

Additional work on interaction effects in a model of medical care use was conducted by Mutran and Ferraro (1988). Their study, using data from a low-income aged subsample of the 1973 Survey of the Low-Income Aged and Disabled (SLIAD), focused on the additive and interactive effects of gender and race in medical care use. Although women are likely to be more frequent users of physician services than men, age was found to act as an "equalizer" of physician contacts among men and women. However, they found evidence that men and women, as well as whites and non-whites, differ in the process that leads them to a physician. "Race and income differentially influenced the assessment of health of men and women; however, men who assessed their health as poor were more likely to see a physician than were women who assessed their health as poor" (p. S169). Further studies are needed, with sufficient numbers of black elderly subjects, to explore the interactions that exist by race.

After examining the issue of the limited ability of large-scale multivariable surveys to explain variance in the use of physician's services among the general population, Mechanic (1979) concluded that one of the major reasons for the problem was that cross-sectional data is unable to measure the dynamic processes involved in the decision to seek care. Based on this conclusion Eve (1988) attempted to increase the amount of variance explained by the behavioral model by including longitudinal measures of two predictors of use of services: a) past health status; and, b) previous use of health care services. The study included 1,894 older women who participated in the Social Security Administration's Longitudinal Retirement History Survey (conducted from 1969 to 1979). Eve (1988) hypothesized that information of past health status and past use of health care services will increase the predictability of the Andersen model. Measures of previous use of health care services were more strongly related to current use of health care services than were measures of previous health status. These results are in keeping with the work of Mossey, Havens and Wolinsky (1989) who found that most older individuals are consistent from year to year in their use of physician care. Inclusion of previous use and previous health status nearly doubled the amount of variance explained using current predictors only. In this study the number of physician visits is truncated (from a maximum of 365 to 21 or more), however, contact is not differentiated from volume of services.

Despite the quantity and quality of the research conducted thus far, relatively little is known about the utilization behaviors of black elderly. The studies cited, typical of the majority of studies in utilization research, include aged blacks and other minorities in one category designated as 'nonwhite' or have such a small proportion of elderly blacks in the study as to render the results meaningless. As a result, relatively little empirical knowledge exists regarding the importance of various predictive variables in determining use among black elderly. To address this problem, Keith and Jones (1990) used data from the 1975 National Survey of the Aged, a probability sample of noninstitutionalized persons aged 65 and older, to examine some of the methodological and substantive issues raised in the area of race and utilization. Included in the sample were 1,969 whites and 416 blacks. Their study examined factors important in determining health care use within the two groups and the ability of the behavioral model to explain utilization by blacks and white elders. They estimated separate models for blacks and whites with the goal of isolating differential patterns of utilization and detection of possible interaction effects. With the probability of having any physician contact as the outcome, they found that among elderly blacks, being widowed, living alone, being in the labor force, place of residence and perceived health status are significantly associated with having physician contact. While sex, education, living alone, having private health insurance, and perceived health status affect the probability that white elders see a physician. Living alone and perceived health status are the only two variables significant for both blacks and whites. Although this study lends support to differences in predictors of utilization for the two groups further research is indicated. First, an analysis of racial differences in the volume of services, an issue not addressed by this study, is needed. Second, this study used data from the mid 1970's; examination of racial differences with more recent data would be useful given changes in Medicare. Third, recent studies (Escarce et al., 1993; Becker et al., 1993; Whittle et al., 1993) have pointed to differences in the content of services received by blacks and whites. It is not clear whether this is attributed to discrimination within the delivery system or whether differential attitudes toward the system deter elderly blacks from seeking needed medical care.

Empirical Literature Summary

The overview of studies examining health care use by elderly people highlights several areas needing further investigation. First, Wan (1989) argues that "need-for-care is an underlying or latent construct that may be measured by multiple correlated instrumental variables, including both objective and subjective measures of health care needs and health status" (p.63). Objective indicators more accurately reflect the physiological dimension of health status while subjective indicators more accurately reflect the individual's perception of and response to his or her physiological state (Shanas and Maddox, 1985). Therefore, according to Wan, the objective indicators can be considered to measure 'need' for health care, whereas subjective indicators can be said to measure 'demand' for health care. It then follows that objective and subjective measures would predict different types and amounts of health care utilization. Wan (1989) urges the development of a measurement model based on subjective and objective indicators and the evaluation of such a model using linear structural relationships (LISRL) approach.

Second, unit of analysis, or the way in which the use of health care services is measured and defined is important. Contact measures indicate whether or not a particular service was used during a defined period of time. This measure focuses more on access to health care rather than on consumption, accordingly, one would expect that indicators of contact would differ from indicators of consumption (Wolinsky, 1990). Volume measures indicate how many services are used during a given time period. Typically, this is given as number of physician visits during the year preceding data collection. Many researchers recommend that studies of use of health care employ both contact and volume measures (Hulka and Wheat, 1985; Branch and Nemeth, 1985; Penchansky and Thomas, 1981; Wolinsky, 1990).

Third, in his review of the behavioral model Wolinsky (1990) advocates the use of a more "saturated", as opposed to a "limited", model for health care use. This issue was raised earlier in Hulka and Wheat's (1985) work when citing from Hershey and colleagues (1975). In the Hershey study the structure of the model and significance of particular variables varied as a function of the number and character of the independent variables included in the model. Hulka and Wheat give as an example that gender (i.e., being female) was associated with an increased number of physician visits until health status variables were included. After their inclusion, being female no longer had a significant effect on the number of physician visits. Hershey et al. (1975) advise against modeling utilization with a restricted set of independent variables. Rather they recommend, as does Wolinsky, a full compliment of variables to stabilize the relationships represented by the model (Hulka and Wheat, 1985). This argument is supported by the findings of Evashwick (1984) which determined that predisposing and enabling factors confound the relationship between need-for-care and utilization of services.

Fourth, measures of perceived access and/or attitudinal barriers to utilization need to be included in an analytic model of physician utilization. While enabling characteristics, the lack of which can present access barriers to Medical Care, are often included in the model, the perceptions of access to and attitudes toward medical care have not been included in a model of utilization behavior.

Finally, additional work needs to be done to enhance the understanding of the utility of the behavioral model to a black elderly population. Prior studies have either been limited by small samples or were unable to examine predictors of both contact with and volume of services. The role of race as mediating the relationship between elements of the behavioral model and utilization need to be explored in an analytic model of physician utilization.

III

Conceptual Model and Hypotheses

This chapter contains a description of the conceptual model that underlies this research, and a discussion of related hypotheses. The first section provides an overview of the conceptual model. The next section contains an overview of the hypothesized relationships and rationale behind hypothesized effects, while the remaining section contains a discussion of the significance of the study.

CONCEPTUAL MODEL

The primary focus of this research is to explore the determinants of the propensity to forego needed medical care and the association of delaying behavior with overall physician utilization. The conceptual model selected is based on modifications of the model proposed by Aday and Andersen on Access to Health Care (1974). Figure 3.1 presents a schematic outline of a somewhat reformulated version of their conceptual model. The path diagram depicts domains or groups of (rather than individual) variables. Some of the variables included in the domains of the Andersen model are predicted to have direct effects on the decision to delay needed medical care and on utilization. Other variables will have direct and /or indirect effects on utilization.

It should also be noted that in the Aday and Andersen schema (1974), factors believed to reflect the ability to access care (such as insurance, income, or usual source of care) were included in the model of utilization while the individual's perceptions regarding issues of access and attitudes were not included. The conceptual model in this research is designed to take into account both: 1) the direct effects of the predisposing, enabling and need-for-care factors on physician utilization, and 2) the indirect effects of these variables on physician utilization via delaying behaviors attributed to perceptions about access to and/or attitudes toward medical care.

Figure 3.1: Model of Perceptions of Access Barriers, Attitudinal Barriers and Utilization

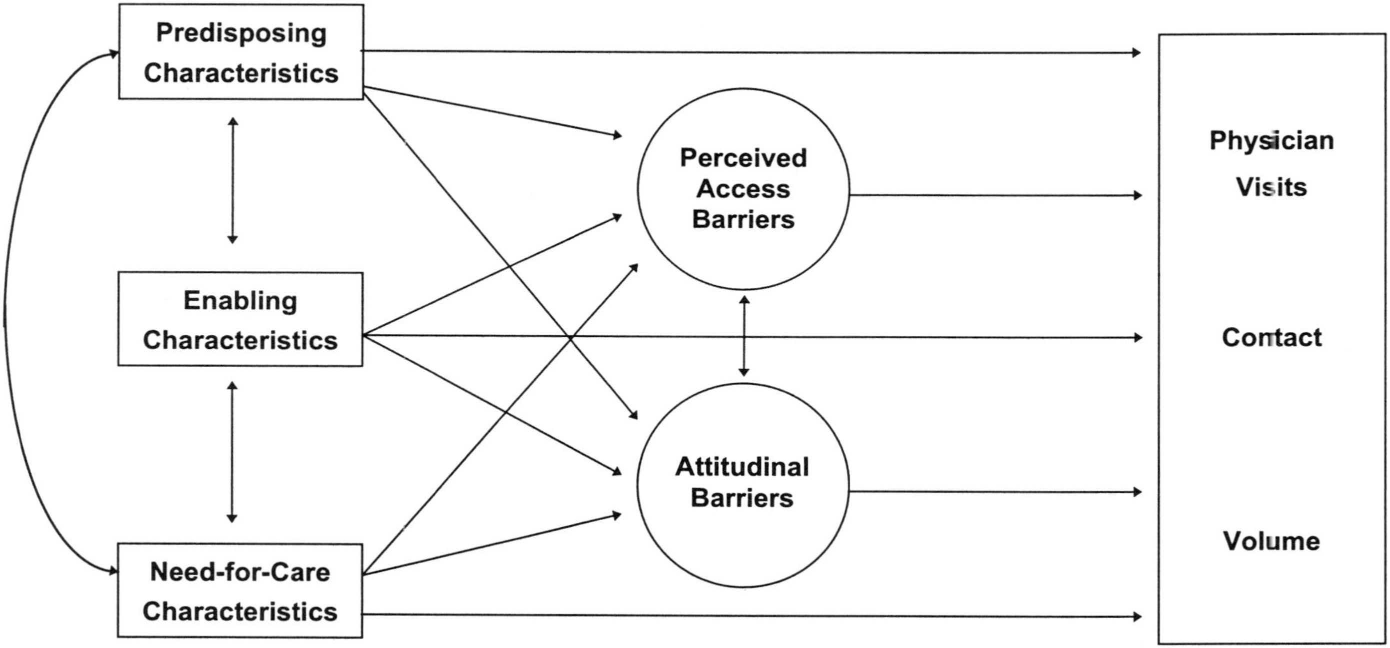

Review of the literature in the previous chapter suggests that variation in the decision to seek and use physician services by elderly people is contingent upon a variety of factors. The framework underlying this research which shape these factors is based on the Andersen behavioral model of health care use. As discussed in the previous chapter, use of physician visits is influenced by elderly individuals' predisposing, enabling and need-for-care characteristics. In the modifications made by this research, these characteristics also influence the propensity to delay medical care. This decision in turn influences the actual use of medical care. In other words, elderly people who report a propensity to delay seeking medical care in response to a need and attribute the delay to access and/or attitudinal barriers use less medical care. In this model, the effects of predisposing, enabling, and need-for-care variables are both direct and indirect; indirect via the perceptions elderly people have about their ability to access care or the perceptions regarding the benefit of a visit.

Table 3.1 summarizes the indicator variables within each domain, used to measure predisposing, enabling and need-for-care characteristics. Predisposing characteristics include age, education, gender, household composition, marital status and race. Enabling characteristics include income, availability of health insurance, usual source of medical care, geographic location of residence, and social support. Self-rated health status, physical function and physical health status are the variables used to measure need for medical care.

Delaying medical care because of perceived barriers of access is defined as putting off or neglecting to seek medical care often because of concerns with cost, transportation difficulties or not knowing where to go for care. While delaying because of attitudinal barriers is defined as regularly putting off or neglecting to seek care because of judging the problem to be self-limiting (getting better without intervention) and/or questioning the efficacy of a physician visit (reporting that going to the doctor would not do any good).

Table 3.1 : Indicator Variables Listed by Domain

Predisposing	Enabling	Need for Care
Age	Income	Self-Rated Health
Education	Health Insurance	Physical Function
Race	Social Support	Physical Health Status
Household Composition	Geographic Location	
Marital Status	Usual Source of Medical Care	
Gender		

HYPOTHESES

Predisposing, Enabling and Need-for-Care Characteristics and Delaying Medical Care

This research builds on the work of Branch and Nemeth (1985), and relies on their findings regarding elderly who fail to seek medical care as the basis for the hypothesized relationships presented here. The hypothesized direction of association between predisposing, enabling and need-for-care characteristics and the likelihood of delaying needed medical care because of access and/or attitudinal barriers is summarized in Tables 3.2 and 3.3. It is hypothesized that the following characteristics are associated with an increase in the likelihood of delaying needed medical care because of perceived access barriers (concern with cost, transportation or distance, or being unsure where to seek care): increased age, living alone, having no usual source of medical care, having no additional insurance to Medicare, and living in a rural county. The following characteristics are predicted to decrease the likelihood of delaying needed medical care because of access barriers: being male (with the exception of knowing where to seek medical care, males should be less likely to encounter financial or transportation difficulties), being married, increased income, having health insurance in addition to Medicare, and worsening health status (as health status decreases the likelihood of being unsure where to go decreases).

The following characteristics are predicted to be associated with an increase in the likelihood of delaying medical care because of perceived attitudinal barriers: increased age, being male, and having no usual source of medical care. Characteristics predicted to be associated with a decrease in the likelihood include: increased education, living alone, being married, having health insurance in addition to Medicare, having a private or public source of care and poorer health status. Relationships represented by question marks indicate areas in the literature where guidance for predicting direction of association is insufficient.

Table 3.2: Hypothesized relationships between subject characteristics and delaying medical care because of perceived access barriers.

Subject Characteristic	Concern with Cost of Visit	Transportation or Distance Difficulties	Unsure of Where to Go
Predisposing			
Age	+	+	?
Education	-	-	
Gender (Male=1)	-	-	+
Household Composition (living alone=1)	+	+	+
Marital Status (married=1)	?	?	?
Race (Black=1)	?	?	?
Enabling			
Income	-	-	-
Health Insurance	-	-	-
Usual Source of Care			
Private	+	+	-
Public	-	?	-
None	+	?	+
Social Support			
Network	-	-	-
Instrumental	-	-	-
Rural Residence	?	+	?
Need-for-Care			
Self-Rated Health	+	+	-
Physical Function	+	+	-
Illness Index	+	+	-

Table 3.3: Hypothesized relationships between subject characteristics and delaying medical care because of attitudinal barriers.

Subject Characteristic	Problem Will Resolve by Itself	Going Won't Do Any Good
Predisposing		
Age	+	+
Education	?	+
Gender (Male=1)	?	-
Household Composition (living alone=1)	-	-
Marital Status (married=1)	?	
Race (Black=1)	?	?
Enabling		
Income	?	?
Health Insurance	-	-
Usual Source of Care		
Private	+	+
Public	-	?
None	+	?
Social Support		
Network	-	-
Instrumental	-	-
Rural Residence	?	+
Need-for-Care		
Self-Rated Health	+	+
Physical Function	+	+
Illness Index	+	+

Delaying Needed Medical Care and Physician Utilization

In their study of elderly people who fail to visit physicians, Branch and Nemeth (1985) found that elders who delay medical care because of attributing health problems to age were more likely to be out of annual physician contact, while elders who delay medical care because of appointment difficulties had increased reported frequencies of physician visits. It seems that those who experience the most frustration with seeking medical care (such as getting an appointment or having transportation difficulties) are those who use the system most often. On the other hand, elderly people who doubt the seriousness of their symptoms or the ability of physicians to do anything about their symptoms are more likely to avoid going altogether. Based on this research, the following hypotheses predict the direction of association between indicators of delay in medical care and overall physician use:

H1: Delaying medical care because of concern with cost or transportation difficulties will not alter the likelihood of having contact with a physician. However, delaying medical care because of being unsure of where to go for care will be associated with a decrease in the likelihood of having had contact with a physician during the preceding twelve months.

H2: Delaying medical care because of perceived access *barriers* (concern with cost, transportation difficulties or being unsure where to go for care) will be associated with a reduction in overall volume of physician visits among users of care.

H3: Delaying medical care because of *attitudinal barriers* will be associated with a decrease in the likelihood of having had any contact with a physician during the preceding twelve months.

H4: Delaying medical care because of *attitudinal barriers* will be associated with a reduction in overall volume of physician visits among users of care.

These hypotheses are summarized below in Table 3.4.

Table 3.4: Hypothesized effect of delaying medical care because of perceived access and/or attitudinal barriers on physician visits.

Variable	NO Physician Contact During the Preceding 12 Months	Number of Physician Visits Among Users of Care
H1 and H2: **Access Barriers**		
Concern with Cost	?	-
Transportation	?	-
Unsure of where to go for care	+	-
H3 and H4: **Attitudinal Barriers**		
Problem will resolve without intervention	+	-
Going to the doctor won't do any good	+	-

Predisposing, Enabling and Need-for-Care Characteristics and Physician Visits

Table 3.5 summarizes the effects of predisposing, enabling and need for care characteristics and the likelihood of reporting *any* contact with a physician during the preceding 12 months, as well as the number of physician visits among users of care (see the Appendix for rationale behind hypothesized effects in Table 3.5). Characteristics associated with an increase in the likelihood of having no physician contact include: being male and having no usual source of care. Characteristics predicted to decrease the likelihood of having no contact with a physician include: age, education, living alone, being married, income, having health insurance supplementary to Medicare, having a usual source of care (either private or public), and poorer health status.

Characteristics predicted to increase the volume of physician visits among users of care include: age, living alone, income, health insurance, usual source of care, and poorer health status. The following characteristics are predicted to decrease the volume of physician visits: being male and having no usual source of medical care.

Health Status, Delaying Medical Care and Physician Visits

Based on the work of Bekanovic, Telesky and Reeder (1981), Krause (1990) hypothesized that elderly persons' belief in the efficacy of medical care will increase as symptoms of physical illness intensify. According to Krause:

> " . . . this hypothesis recognizes that older adults may believe that they are capable of handling relatively minor symptoms on their own, whereas they may value the expertise and technology provided in formal care settings in those instances where symptoms become more severe or life threatening (p. 237)."

Accordingly,

> H5: As the level of health status decreases (illness level increases) the likelihood of delaying medical care because of attitudinal barriers will decrease and the utilization of physician visits will increase.

Social Support, Delaying Medical Care and Physician Visits

The behavioral model predicts that individuals' decision to seek medical care is determined in part by the attitudes of members of their social network (Krause, 1990). If significant others value medical care then they will encourage the elderly individual to obtain care when a need arises and provide instrumental support which would enable the individual to seek care (such as transportation or financial assistance). On the other hand, if members of one's social network distrust medical care or doubt its effectiveness, then they will discourage the individual from seeking medical care or will be less likely to provide the instrumental support which would enable the individual to overcome access barriers.

Six measures of social support are used in the proposed analysis, two of which (household composition, i.e., whether an individual lives alone, and marital status), have been used by other investigators (Evashwick et al., 1984), and are included as a predisposing characteristic. The other four include: 1) two measures of the individual's network (availability of friends and availability of family); and, 2) two measures of instrumental support (assistance with illness and assistance with transportation). These are included as enabling characteristics.

Berkanovic and colleagues (1981) contend that under threat of illness individuals begin to seek information and support from their network or social contacts. They hypothesized that "highly interdependent 'strong tie' networks, where there is consultation with few persons, lead to delay behaviors since group opinion tends to be uniform and tends to support the individual to stay well. 'Weak tie' networks with diverse contacts may provide confusing and disparate information which causes an individual to seek professional advice sooner" (Berkanovic et al., 1981; p. 698). However, increased support from network was found to be associated with an increase in the likelihood of seeking medical care for symptoms and network size had no effect on the likelihood of seeking care. In addition, people who reported that their friends would help in time of need were more likely to see a physician for symptoms.

Therefore, it is hypothesized that:

H6: The availability of social support (particularly receiving assistance from others) will be associated with a decrease in the likelihood of delaying medical care because of perceived access barriers.

H7: The availability of social support (particularly receiving assistance from others) will be associated with an increase in the likelihood of having one or more visits to a physician over the course of a year, and an increase in the volume of services among users of care.

The effect of social support on delaying behaviors attributed to attitudinal barriers can only be fully understood if the attitudes of the individuals comprising the support network is known. Attitudes toward the health care system on the part of the subject's support network are not available here.

Race and the Relationship Between Delaying Medical Care and Physician Visits

The review of the literature pointed to the significance of race as a potential modifier of the relationship between measures of access and utilization. The role of race in the decision to delay medical care, the reasons for delay, and the effect of a propensity to delay on physician visits are not known. Race has been found to exacerbate the impact of other barriers to care (Escarce et al., 1993), however, perceptions of access and attitudes toward medical care are not well understood.

Elderly blacks have more extensive family systems than elderly whites (Taylor, 1985), and black families are more involved than white families in exchanges of help across generations (Mutran, 1985). Additionally, a broader network of non-kin appears to occupy a more central position in black social support networks (Chatters, Taylor and Jackson, 1986), providing elderly blacks with a more extensive network of family and friends who they can call on when they have problems (Ulbrich and Bradsher, 1993).

Therefore,

H8: Race will modify the relationship between predisposing, enabling and need-for-care characteristics and delay in seeking medical care and utilization.

SIGNIFICANCE OF THE STUDY

Considering the abundance of research on the topic of health care utilization by the elderly, it is appropriate to ask what this study can contribute to the literature. It is the author's belief that this study is of both methodological and policy significance. Below is a summary of the ways in which this work contributes to the field:

Methodological Significance. This study explores the usefulness of including attitudinal and perceived access barriers to care in a model of health care utilization in an older population thereby enhancing the utility of Andersen's health behavior model in this population. Furthermore, incorporating a construct pertaining to beliefs about the efficacy of medical care provides some overlap between the health behavior and health beliefs models, as well as a common theme to bind them together.

Additionally, some investigators (for example Wan, 1989; Wolinsky, 1990) have proposed using methods such as two-staged least squares and simultaneous equations estimations in an attempt to increase the predictability of the Andersen model in the elderly population. This study contributes methodologically by examining both direct and indirect effects of individual characteristics on utilization of physician services.

This study also explores the importance of including interaction terms between race and predisposing, enabling and need-for-care characteristics in a model of health care utilization.

Policy Significance. There is a concern on the part of investigators and policy makers that "persistent, and sometimes, substantial, differences continue to exist in the quality of health among Americans" (American Medical Association, Council on Ethical and Judicial Affairs, 1990; p. 2344), particularly between minorities, such as African-Americans, and whites. While racial disparities in treatment decisions for whites and African-Americans have been noted (see for example, Escarce et al., 1993; Yergan et al., 1987), this study contributes to the understanding of racial differences in *perceptions* of barriers to access. Previous studies suggest, that in a younger population, blacks are more likely to delay medical care, as compared with whites (Weissman et al., 1991). This study contributes to policy by its investigation of the frequency of delay in seeking medical care among elderly blacks and elderly whites, whether this delay is attributed to access or to attitudinal barriers, and the effect of delay on the utilization of medical care by both groups. If, despite the nearly universal health care coverage provided for elders by Medicare, elderly African-Americans perceive significant deterrents to their ability to access medical care, and this in turn influences their utilization of medical care, then this knowledge is relevant for the formation of policy.

As policy makers debate the future of the American health care system, this research contributes to the debate by furthering the understanding of health care utilization by a segment of the population of older adults with nearly universal health insurance coverage (Medicare), and the role of insurance supplementary to baseline coverage on utilization.

IV

Research Design and Methodology

The discussion of research design begins with sample description and data source. Variables to be included in the analysis are then defined followed by specification of the empirical model to be estimated along with an overview of statistical issues related to analysis and analytic techniques used to measure determinants of the propensity to delay needed medical care and its association with use of physician care.

SAMPLE AND DATA SOURCE

In 1980 the Epidemiology, Demography and Biometry Program (EDBP) at the National Institute on Aging (NIA) initiated a project entitled "The Establishment of Populations for Epidemiologic Studies of the Elderly" (EPESE). Initially, the EPESE project included studies of noninstitutionalized elderly persons in three communities: East Boston, Massachusetts; Iowa and Washington Counties, Iowa; and New Haven, Connecticut (Cornoni-Huntley et al., 1986). In 1984 a fourth site was initiated in a five county area surrounding Durham, North Carolina. The goal of this latter location was to provide information on black elderly (Cornoni-Huntley et al., 1990).

This study is a secondary analysis of baseline data from the Piedmont Health Survey of the Elderly (PHSE), the Durham site of the EPESE project. The North Carolina sample consists of 4,162 persons aged 65 and older from five contiguous counties in North Carolina. Figure 4.1 provides a map of the geographic study area which includes Durham, Granville, Vance, Warren and Franklin Counties located in the Piedmont region of North Carolina.

The sample was obtained using a four-stage stratified probability sampling design. In the first stage, primary sampling units consisting of 450 zones of approximately equal population size were selected from the survey area. In the second stage, one listing area was selected from each zone. Within the listing area, all households were enumerated. The third stage involved the selection of households within listing areas. At the fourth stage, one person aged 65 years or older was selected from each eligible household. One of the primary missions of the EPESE project is an examination of differences in health between black and white elderly community residents. Consequently, blacks were intentionally over-sampled so that they represented 55 percent of the selected sample.

Of 5,223 persons who were eligible for the study 4,162 agreed to be interviewed, yielding an 80 percent response rate. Sample members deleted from this study include subjects for whom a proxy interview was conducted and for whom data on delaying medical care are not available, and respondents who were neither black nor white.

Figure 4.1: Geographic Study Area

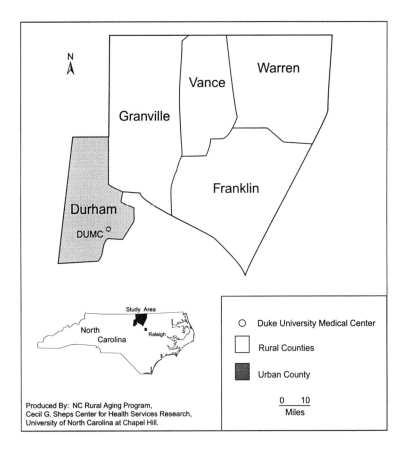

VARIABLE DEFINITION

Variables included in the analysis were selected because of their correspondence to the model and because previous research related them to health service use among elderly people. The variables were aggregated with the Andersen model as a framework. The independent variables, grouped as predisposing, enabling and need-for-care factors, and dependent variables (delaying needed medical care and physician visits), are defined in the following section. Table 4.1 provides a summary of the explanatory variables included in the analysis, their definition and coding, while Table 4.2 provides the same for the dependent variables.

Predisposing Characteristics

There are 6 measures of predisposing characteristics. These include age, gender, race, household composition, marital status and education. Each of these variables is defined below.

Age (AGE). This is a continuous variable and is defined as age of the subject, in years.

Education (EDUC). A continuous variable defined as number of years in school. In Wolinsky and Johnson's (1991) analysis of utilization data from the Longitudinal Study on Aging, education was included as a continuous variable defined as actual number of years of education. They found that education was positively associated with an increase in the number of physician visits among those who had at least one visit but had no effect on physician contact. This analysis follows the Wolinsky and Johnson definition of education.

Gender (MALE). The referent category for gender is female and the variable is coded as '1' = male and '0' = female.

Household Composition (ALONE). A subject living alone is coded as '1' and a subject living with others is coded as '0'.

Race. Comparisons of interest in this analysis are between African-American and Caucasian elderly. The former is coded as '1' and the latter as '0'.

Marital Status. A currently married subject is coded as '1' while a subject not currently married is coded as '0'.

Table 4.1: Measurement and Operational Definition of Explanatory Variables

VARIABLE	MEASUREMENT	OPERATIONAL DEFINITION
Predisposing		
Age	Interval	Age of subject
Gender	Dichotomous	'1' = male; '0' = female
Race	Dichotomous	'1' = Black; '0' = White
Education	Interval	Years of schooling
Marital Status	Dichotomous	'1' = married '0' = not married
Living Alone	Dichotomous	'1' = lives alone '0' = lives with others
Enabling		
Income	Categorical - included in the analysis as dummy variables; referent category 5,000.	Annual personal income from all sources categorized into: 5,000 $5-9,999 $10-19,999 $20,000 or more
Health Insurance	Categorical - included in the analysis as a series of dummy variable with the referent category being Medicare insurance only.	Categories include: Medicare only Medicare and private supplementary insurance Medicaid Health Maintenance Organization
Usual Source of Medical Care	Categorical - defining place of care and included in the analysis as dummy variables with the referent category private physician office.	Categories include: Private physician office Clinic (e.g., clinic, OPD) No usual place
Social support: Network	Dichotomous - two measures; one measuring availability of a relative, the other measures the availability of a friend	Availability of relative to rely on '1' = yes; '0' = no Availability of friend to rely on '1' = yes; '0' = no

Table 4.1 continued

VARIABLE	MEASUREMENT	OPERATIONAL DEFINITION
Instrumental	Dichotomous - two measures; one measures assistance with illness, the other assistance with transportation.	Assistance when ill '1' = yes; '0' = no Assistance with transportation '1' = yes; '0' = no
Geographic location	Dichotomous	'1' = Rural, defined as residing in Warren, Granville, Vance and Franklin counties. '0' = Urban, defined as residing in Durham County.
Need-for-Care		
Self-Rated Health	Categorical - included in the analysis as a series of dummy variables with the referent category being excellent/good health.	Assessed as excellent, good, fair or poor.Excellent and good categories were collapsed leaving three categories: excellent/good, fair and poor.
Disability	Dichotomous	'1' = requiring assistance in performing at least one of 7 activity of daily living. '0' = independent in all 7 items.
Illness Index	Categorical - included in the analysis as dummy variables with the referent category being 'good health'; the other two categories are fair and poor health.	Measures the presence and severity of chronic illness including hypertension, diabetes, heart disease and cancer.Categories include: good health - score 0-21 fair health -score 22-54 poor health -score 55 +

Enabling Characteristics

The five measures of enabling characteristics are defined below. They include income, health insurance, usual source of medical care, geographic location and social support. In a study by Wolinsky and Johnson (1991) social support was included as a predisposing variable. In the analyses presented here social support is defined as an enabling characteristic because of the instrumental and psychological support which can facilitate care seeking and utilization of services.

Income. The income variable includes reported and imputed income data. Annual personal income is divided into 4 categories including: less than $5,000 ; $5,000-9,999; $10,000-19,999; and $20,000 or more. Results of bivariate relationships between income and dependent variables (see Chapter IV) determined that it would be best to include income as dummy variables when modeling perceptions and utilization. Coding income as a series of dummy variables does not impose any assumptions on the relationship between income and the dependent variable of interest. On the other hand, including income in the analysis as an ordinal variable assumes that the impact of the variable is constant from one income level to another.

Health Insurance. Categories of health insurance include: Medicare only (MEDICARE); Medicaid (MEDICAID); Supplementary insurance to Medicare (MEDIGAP); and health maintenance organization (HMO). These are included in the analysis as a series of dummy variables with the referent category being Medicare only. Medicare recipients without supplementary policies are less likely to seek medical care or advice as compared with those with private supplementary insurance (Millman, 1993, p. 113). These measures of health insurance capture key elements of coverage status (i.e., private and public welfare transfer) accordingly, the referent category Medicare only provides a comparison of added benefits to Medicare on care seeking behaviors and use of services.

Usual Source of Medical Care. Participants in the Piedmont Health Survey were asked "When you want help with or care for a (physical) health problem, where do you usually go?" If the response was 'nowhere' or 'no usual place' subjects were skipped to the next question, however, if a usual source was given respondents were asked to name the physician or the practice site. Responses were then coded under categories that include: physician or clinic, not hospital based; physician or clinic, hospital based; and other location. For the purposes of these analyses, responses were categorized as: 1) Private - subjects who name as their usual source of care a private physician office either hospital or not hospital based; 2) Clinic - subjects who name as their usual source of care a public clinic or outpatient clinic; 3) no usual place - subjects who state that they go 'nowhere', have no usual place, or name an urgent clinic, emergency clinic or emergency room as their usual source of care. These categories are included in the analysis as dummy variables with the referent category being 'private'.

Geographic Location (RURAL). Geographic location is determined by the study participant's county of residence. Residents of Durham County were designated as living in the urban location and coded as '0', while residents of Warren, Granville, Vance and Franklin Counties were designated as living in a rural locale and coded as '1'.

Social Support. Four questionnaire items were used to measure social support. They include the following:

1. Number of relatives the subject feels close to or can call on for help.

2. Number of friends, other than family, the subject feels close to or can call on for help.

3. Whether assistance was received for illness.

4. Whether assistance was received for transportation.

Together, these four items provide a measure of two aspects of social support. The first two items measure the extent of an individual's network and availability of someone in the network to whom the older adult can turn to for support and/or advice. Items 3 and 4 provide a measure of instrumental support received, not support needed. Note that the each item is dichotomized and included in the analysis as no support ('1') versus any support ('0').

Need-for-Care Characteristics

Three measures of need-for-care are included: self-rated health status, physical function, and the presence of chronic illness.

Self-rated health status. To assess self-rated health status respondents were asked: "Overall, how would you rate your health - as excellent, good, fair or poor?" Following Wolinsky, Arnold and Nallapati's (1988) suggestion, excellent and good responses are collapsed, indicating good self perceived health. However, fair or poor responses are examined as separate categories in bivariate analysis.

Physical Function. Katz and colleagues (1963) developed a Guttman scale measuring the ability to perform activities of daily living (ADL). The measure calls for a dichotomous rating of the following items: bathing, dressing, going to the toilet, transferring, continence and feeding. One point is given for each item of dependency. This is one of the best known and most carefully studied measures of ADL (Kane and Kane, 1980). In the EPESE data participants were asked the following items from the Katz scale:

> "Now I'm going to ask you some questions about the kind of help you need to do things:
>
> 1. walking across a small room? (not a Katz item)
>
> 2. bathing? (either a sponge bath, tub bath, or shower)
>
> 3. personal grooming like brushing hair, brushing teeth, or washing face?
>
> 4. dressing? (like putting on a shirt, buttoning and zipping, or putting on shoes)
>
> 5. eating ? (like holding a fork, cutting food, or drinking from a glass)
>
> 6. getting from a bed to a chair?
>
> 7. using the toilet?"

Because this is a sample of community residents it is likely that only a small proportion of older adults would be dependent in these activities of daily living. Consequently, this variable is coded as '1' indicating *any* disability in any of the activities listed and '0' indicating no difficulty.

*Physical Health Status (*Illness Index). The PHSE researchers developed a simple, valid, reliable and readily usable measure of the physical health status of PHSE participants (Fillenbaum et al., 1993). Information was gathered from subjects on five common health conditions: heart problems, hypertension, diabetes, stroke and cancer. If the condition was present, a series of questions followed to determine the level of severity. Where measurements were readily feasible, as in determining blood pressure or the presence of glucose or protein in the urine, those measurements were obtained. A listing of current medications was obtained so that whether a medication was taken for a particular disorder was known. For each condition, a panel of physicians was asked to indicate the item's impact on health. For any one condition scores could range from 0 (condition absent) to 68. As indicated below, a scoring algorithm was devised with total possible scores ranging from 0 to 331 with higher scores reflecting a greater severity of illness.

	Actual Scoring Range
Heart condition	0 - 64
Hypertension	0 - 67
Diabetes	0 - 66
Stroke	0 - 65
Cancer	0 - 69
Total Possible	0 - 331

To assess validity, the scale was compared to other known indicators of health such as: health service use, self-rated health, functional status, and socioeconomic status. Because of the skewed distribution of the scale, three categories were created with cut-off at the 33 and the 67 percentiles so that they had an indication of good, fair and poor health. In general, they found that those in poorer health on the illness index made greater use of health services, had poorer self-rated health and were more likely to be functionally impaired. The internal validity the scale was checked by means of Cronbach's alpha with a value of .94 obtained on this measure. Reliability of this measure remains to be determined.

While the index includes some of the conditions which are among the leading causes of death in this population, it should be noted that other chronic conditions prevalent among the elderly, arthritis for example, which motivate an individual to seek medical care are not represented. Nor does the scale include information on hearing or vision. This scale was not developed as a measure of health. Rather, its value lies in its use as a control for physical health status so that other relationships of interest can be explored.

A three level categorical variable was constructed by the PHSE study. These were: a) good health - score ranged from 0 to 21; b) fair health - score ranged from 22 to 54; and, c) poor health - score included 55 and over. To enhance consistency among users of data from the PHSE, this scoring algorithm was adopted for this study.

Delaying Needed Medical Care

All non-proxy respondents were asked (see Table 4.2): "How often do you put off or neglect going to the doctor when you feel that you really should go?" 'Never', 'Once in a While', or 'Quite Often'.

Subjects reporting any delay were then asked about their reasons:

"I'll read some reasons why some people don't go to the doctor when they think they really should. Which ones are reasons why you sometimes haven't gone to the doctor?

1) Did you think that the problem would get better by itself? (yes, no)

2) Were you concerned about the cost? (yes, no)

3) Were you unsure about where to go for help? (yes, no)

4) Did you think that going to the doctor wouldn't do any good? (yes, no)

5) Was it too difficult to go to the doctor because of distance or transportation problems? (yes, no)

These questions are similar to those used by national surveys of randomly selected samples of ambulatory populations, which also relied on self-reports to assess patients' decisions to seek care (for example, the National Medical Care Utilization and Expenditure Survey). Significant correlation between self-reported and actual delay in seeking care have been reported in previous studies (Weissman et al., 1991).

Delaying needed medical care is defined as postponing or neglecting to seek care often, when an individual thinks she really should go, for one of the five reasons given above. Need is determined by the individual's perception of need for a physician visit. This delineation results in five variables representing two conceptual categories and defined as:

1) Reported delay of needed medical care attributed to perceived access barriers:

   a. concern with cost (COST)
   b. distance or lack of transportation (NOTRANS)
   c. being unsure as to where to go for medical care (WHERE)

Table 4.2: Measurement and Operational Definition of
Dependent Variables

VARIABLE	MEASUREMENT	PERATIONAL DEFINITION
Delay:		
Failure to seek needed medical care attributed to perceived access barriers:		
Concern with cost	Dichotomous	1 = delaying needed care often because of cost.
		0 = not delaying for this reason.
Problems with distance or transportation	Dichotomous	1 = delaying needed care often because for this reason.
		0 = not delaying for this reason.
Not knowing where to go for care	Dichotomous	1 = delaying needed care often for this reason.
		0 = not delaying for this reason.
Failure to seek needed medical care attributed to attitudinal barriers:		
Attributed to the belief that the problem is self limiting.	Dichotomous	1 = delaying needed care often because of the belief that the problem would get better by itself.
		0 = not delaying for this reason.
Attributed to the belief that intervention would not do any good.	Dichotomous	1 = delaying needed care often because of the belief that going would not do any good.
		0 = not delaying for this reason.
Physician Visits		
Volume of visits among users of care	Interval	Number of physician visits for those having at least 1 visit truncated with 12 or more visits equaling 12.

2) Reported delay of needed medical care attributed to attitudinal barriers:

    a. seeing a doctor won't do any good (NOGOOD)
    b. the problem will get better by itself (BETTER)

For each of these measures a '1' indicates that the subject delayed needed medical care for this reason while a '0' indicates that the subject did not.

Reasons for delay are not mutually exclusive categories. An affirmative response could be given to as many of the reasons as apply. Consequently, these categories cannot be analyzed as a multinomial dependent variable. Five models are estimated with each model examining the determinants of delaying needed medical care attributed to a particular reason.

In the context of this investigation, need for medical care is presumed when an individual reports a perceived need to visit a physician. Whether the individual subsequently acts, however, is influenced by perceptions regarding the effectiveness of action and barriers to action.

Physician Visits

Following the suggestion of Branch and Nemeth (1985), physician visits are defined as two separate outcome variables: contact and volume of services. First, physician visits were dichotomized into no visits during the 12 months preceding the interview versus one or more visits. Second, physician visits were defined as the number of physician visits among users of service (Branch and Nemeth, 1985). Because the number of reported visits often exhibits marked skewness and kurtosis, this study followed Wolinsky and Coe's (1984) recommendation that truncated or transformed variables be used to minimize the distortion caused by the few respondents with extremely high use of health physician visits. Truncation rather than transformation was used because of ease of interpretation. Wolinsky and Coe recommend that the truncation be set where the tails of the distributions become flat, generally with only 5 percent of the sample of respondents exceeding the criterion level. The distribution of this variable was examined and cutoff established so that number of visits ranged from 1 to 12.

Members Excluded from the Study

The Piedmont Health Survey of the Elderly included 4,162 persons, however, the analyses included here included 3,746 persons. Proxy respondents (n=169), missing data for any of the seven dependent variables (n=221), and participants who were neither white nor black (n=26) were dropped from the analysis. Decisions to drop members from the analysis were made for the following reasons: 1) proxy respondents were not asked questions about perceptions of access or delay decisions, 2) data for outcome variables cannot be imputed and, 3) there were too few subjects who were neither white nor black to constitute a meaningful category.

OVERVIEW OF THE ANALYSIS STRATEGY

The analysis begins with a discussion of descriptive statistics, bivariate relationships, and multivariable modeling. This is followed by a discussion of the analytic strategy regarding the role of race as mediating the relationships of interest, as well as a discussion of missing data and significance testing. A presentation of the empirical models are provided followed by estimation techniques.

Descriptive Statistics

Descriptive statistics employed for the various dependent and independent variables depended on whether the variable was continuous or categorical. Univariate analysis for the continuous variables included an examination of central tendency (means, medians), variation (range, variance and standard deviation), distribution and plots (e.g. histogram, stem and leaf, box and normal probability). An examination of frequencies and plots (bar graphs) were included in the univariate analysis of categorical variables.

Bivariate Analysis

The relationship between each of the predisposing, enabling and need for care variables and the outcome variables were evaluated one variable at a time. The strategy for assessing the association between each independent and dependent variables was as follows (Garrett, 1993): a) the Pearson Chi-square test was used to evaluate the association between each of the categorical independent variables and the dichotomous dependent variables; b) a two sample t-test compared means between two groups for variables where the outcome was continuous (number of physician visits) and the independent variable had only two categories; c) the association between the continuous dependent variable and independent variables with more than two categories was assessed using a one-way analysis of variance (ANOVA) with an F statistic estimated for the relationships under study; finally d) the sample was then stratified by race and adjusted and crude odds ratios were compared and significant interactions were noted.

Multivariate Modeling

There are two overall goals of the empirical modeling. First, the analysis models the influence of predisposing, enabling and need for care attributes of the individual on the likelihood of delaying needed medical care for reasons of cost (COST), transportation (NOTRANS), not knowing where to go (WHERE), believing the problem will get better by itself (BETTER), and believing that a visit would not do any good (NOGOOD). Second, controlling for predisposing, enabling and need-for-care characteristics two models were estimated: 1) The relationship between delaying needed medical care and the likelihood of having had any contact with a physician during the preceding twelve months; and 2) The relationship between delaying needed medical care and the volume of physician visits among users of care. Logistic regression using maximum likelihood techniques (MLE) were used to estimate each of the equations having a dichotomous dependent variable. Ordinary least squares regression (OLS) were used for the equation estimating number of physician visits among users of care. Finally, each model was re-estimated using a technique which provides corrected standard errors by applying weights and adjusting for design effect (see discussion about SUDAAN).

The modeling strategy for each outcome variable included the following steps: a) estimation of a full model (with all variables including interaction terms); b) attempts at paring down the model by removing non-significant terms; and, c) evaluating the new model by examining the effect on the coefficients of the remaining variables as well as differences in F-test for the OLS model and log-likelihood ratio test for the logistic models. Steps (b) and (c) were repeated until an acceptable model was obtained.

Modeling the Likelihood of Delaying Needed Medical Care

The five dependent variables in this phase of analysis (COST, NOTRANS, WHERE, BETTER, NOGOOD), modeled as a series of five equations, are qualitative in nature and are represented as dichotomous variables (for example, COST is set equal to '1' for those reporting that they delay needed medical care because of concern with cost and '0' for those not giving this as a reason).

Dichotomous dependent variables violate the assumption of homoscedasticity inherent in ordinary least squares (OLS) regression analysis resulting in coefficient estimates that are consistent and unbiased but not efficient. Consequently, significance testing becomes problematic since the standard errors from such estimations are large (Bollen, lecture notes 1/23/90). Additional OLS estimation problems include 1) predicting outside the 0-1 range of the dependent variable and 2) wrong functional form resulting in potentially inconsistent estimators (Bollen, lecture notes 1/25/90).

In analyzing dichotomous dependent variables the cumulative normal function (or probit) and logistic function (or logit) models are able to provide unbiased and efficient estimates that are inside the 0-1 range of the dependent variable. These two functions are very similar, however, logistic regression provides estimates of odds ratios commonly used in epidemiologic research and are used in the analyses presented here.

Multivariable logistic regression analysis was performed to examine the role of predisposing, enabling and need for care characteristics on the likelihood of delaying needed medical care for each of the five reasons. Odds ratios and confidence intervals were calculated for each variable in the model approximating the relative risk of reporting the propensity to delay needed medical care for subjects in a particular group. All analyses were conducted initially using weights to correct for differing sampling probabilities followed by the use of a statistical package that corrects standard errors for design effect (SUDAAN).

Assumptions of the Logistic Regression Model

The assumptions of the logistic regression model are as follow:

1. Independence of observations.

2. All continuous or ordinal X variables are linear in the log odds of Y.

3. Specification of interaction among the X's, when interaction is present.

The logistic model can be written as:

$$P(Y = 1|\Sigma Xi) = 1/1 + e^{-[a+\Sigma\beta iXi]}$$

and is used to model the risk of an event occurring as a function of various independent variables known or suspected to be related to the outcome (Kleinbaum, Kupper and Morgenstern, 1982). This can be written in the logit as:

$$Logit(Y = 1|\sum Xi) = a + \sum \beta iXi$$

Where Y represents the dichotomous dependent variables and X represents the independent variables. Note that the logistic model is linear in the logit. When exponentiated, each bi can assess change in the odds of event 'y' associated with a one unit increase in Xi, holding all other Xj's constant.

Modeling Utilization of Physician Services

This analysis explores the propensity to delay needed medical care due to perceived access and/or attitudinal barriers and the implications of this behavior on physician utilization. Two models are estimated for the two outcomes defining use of physician services. The first estimates the likelihood of having *no* contact with a physician during the previous twelve months, while the second estimates the volume of physician visits among users of care.

The Likelihood of NO Contact With a Physician

Estimating the likelihood of *no* contact with a physician during the preceding twelve month period, a dichotomous outcome, presents the same violation of homoscedasticity discussed in the previous section. Consequently, using the same logic, this model is estimated using logistic regression.

Volume of Visits Among Users of Care

Volume of services is a continuous outcome variable, and thus, the use of ordinary least squares estimation (OLS) is appropriate. OLS estimator is said to be the best linear unbiased estimator (BLUE) of the beta coefficients when the following assumptions are met: a) independence of observations; b) constant variance; c) approximate normality of the distribution of the error terms; and, d) no specification bias.

Direct and Indirect Effects

Direct effects were determined by the coefficient estimates, while the direction of the indirect effects of the predisposing, enabling and need-for-care factors on use of physician services via delaying behaviors were noted.

Analytic Strategy Regarding the Effects of Race

In this study special attention is given to the role of race as mediating the relationship between predisposing, enabling and need for care variables and delaying needed medical care, and the role of race in the relationship between delaying medical care and utilization. Assessment of the role of race in these relationships is as follows:

1. The bivariate analysis is repeated stratifying for race and results are examined to determine which relationships suggest that the effect varies by race.

2. Multivariate models are estimated initially with race as a dichotomous variable (black versus white elders) including significant interactions (or those of interest) from the bivariate analysis.

3. A likelihood ratio test is then conducted to examine the significance of interaction terms. If the global test is significant then each interaction term is evaluated individually.

4. Significant interactions are reported and summarized.

Missing Data

Missing data for many demographic and composite measures were imputed by PHSE researchers. In order to provide for consistency across analyses in the manner in which missing data are handled, this study used imputed variables and methods available through the PHSE project. The following summarizes the procedure used to deal with missing data (communication with L.R. Landerman[1]). In general, more sophisticated and time-consuming techniques were used for measures with more missing data.

a) *Measures with less than 2 percent missing data*: No imputations were made. The recommendation is to impute the mean (independent variable) or drop cases (dependent variable). Imputing the mean assumes that the data are 'missing completely at random' (MCAR); that respondents and nonrespondents have the same distribution on the variable being imputed. Deviations from MCAR result in biased estimates of the variable mean, however, with 2% or fewer cases missing, bias should be minimal for the sample as a whole (Landerman, 1992).

b)   *Measures with 2 or more, but less than 5 percent missing data*: Deterministic regression methods were employed to assign a regression-based y-hat to substitute for missing values. Deterministic regression imputation can distort the shape of the distribution as well as attenuate the variance of the measure being imputed thereby biasing significance tests. However, as is the case with recoding to the mean, the degree to which the bias occurs depends upon the percent missing. Analysis by the Duke PHSE researchers (Landerman, 1992) indicated that variance attenuation resulting from using deterministic regression methods are minimal for variables with fewer than 5 percent missing.

c)   *Measures with 5 percent or more missing*: Stochastic regression techniques were employed for imputation of these variables (for example, income, marital status, education). This method was also used to impute missing data for composites which had at least 5 percent missing data (for example, amount of social interaction) (for exact method see Landerman, 1992). The regression imputation techniques assume that missing data are MAR - missing at random conditional on the predictors included in the imputation equation. This assumption means "missing and non-missing cases are only randomly different once the predictors in the imputation equation are controlled" (Landerman, 1992; p. 18). Landerman further cautions that in studies "where an imputed measure (especially one with 5 percent or more missing data) serves as a primary research factor or outcome, researchers should examine these predictors carefully and con-sider whether the MAR assumption is appropriate (p. 18)."

Using imputed data present two potential problems: 1) the potentially problematic modeling assumption described above. If there is reason to suspect that nonrespondents may be systematically different from respon-dents on an imputed variable then multiple imputation techniques are available (Rubin, 1987), and 2) bias in significance testing. According to Landerman (1992), a principal source of underestimation is inflated sample size where imputed scores are treated like real data. This results in significance tests which are biased in the direction of increased Type I error. Landerman outlines corrections for this bias which is discussed in the following section.

Significance Testing

The multi-stage, stratified random design of the Duke/EPESE study necessitated the use of analysis weights and adjustments of significance testing in order to permit generalization of findings. In addition, the use of imputed data required adjustment of significance testing[2]. Consequently, initial point estimates and variances were obtained using STATA software[3] which uses proportional weights. However, final runs were conducted using SUDAAN[4] software which corrected standard errors and significance tests, as well as additional corrections for inflated sample size resulting from design effects.

As noted in the previous section, imputation of missing data leads to an underestimation of standard errors resulting from inflated sample size. Landerman (1992) suggests an adjustment where sample size before imputation is used to adjust significance tests. The ratio of this smaller N to the N based on imputed data is then used to adjust standard errors and significance tests. This correction to significance testing results in a likelihood to err on the side of being conservative in order to insure that Type I error rates are not inflated.

INTERNAL VALIDITY

Possible threats to the internal validity of this research include: 1) the possibility of a recursive system with correlated error terms between the equations for delaying needed medical care and physician utilization resulting in a simultaneous equation bias, and 2) recall bias in the measurement of the volume of physician visits. These two issues are addressed below.

Simultaneous Equation Bias

The data used in this study are cross-sectional with the propensity to delay medical care, perceptions of access to medical care and physician visits assessed for the same time period. Consequently, one could argue that an individual's recollection of utilization experience influences perceptions of access and attitudinal barriers to medical care. The model resulting from this argument is illustrated below:

$$Y_{1i} = \beta_{10} + \beta_{12}Y_{2i} + \gamma_{11}X_{1i} + u_{1i}$$

$$Y_{2i} = \beta_{10} + \beta_{21}Y_{1i} + \gamma_{21}X_{1i} + u_{2i}$$

Where, Y_1 (failure to seek needed medical care) and Y_2 (physician visits) are mutually dependent, or endogenous variables, and X_1 (predisposing, enabling and need for care variables) are exogenous, and where u_1 and u_2 are the stochastic disturbance terms. Unless it can be shown that Y_1 is distributed independently of u_1 and Y_2 is distributed independently of u_2 the application of classical OLS or Logistic Regression to these equations individually will lead to inconsistent results (Gujarati, 1988).

If the propensity to forego needed medical care is influenced by unobserved factors reflected the disturbance term for the utilization equations that contribute to use, then the disturbance terms in the first series of equations (estimating the likelihood of failing to seek needed medical care) and the disturbance terms in the second series of equations (estimating the likelihood of contact and volume of physician services) are not independent, and an instrumental variable technique is required for an unbiased estimate of the association between failure to seek medical care and utilization of physician services. However, if the disturbance terms are independent, use of an instrumental variable is less efficient than use of the actual variable.

To summarize, this threat to internal validity can be dealt with in the following two steps:

1. Conduct a Spencer-Berk Test for Endogeneity - Spencer-Berk (Kmenta, 1986) developed a single-equation test of the null hypothesis that a right-hand side variable in an equation is exogenous (i.e., uncorrelated with the error term). This would provide a statistical test indicating whether error terms are correlated.

2. In the event that the Spencer-Berk test is statistically significant then a Two Staged Least Squares (2SLS)[5] estimation would be performed and the beta coefficients from the 2SLS analysis and the single equation method would be compared. If the 2SLS results are similar to those obtained by the logistic ar.d OLS estimations then the logistic and OLS results would be reported since these models are more efficient.

Using this approach is problematic because it is not currently feasible to account for possible endogeneity *and* weight the analysis correcting for sampling and design effects. In addition, 2SLS assumes a continuous dependent variable, and with the exception of the analysis that examines the volume of physician visits among users of care, the dependent variables in this study are dichotomous. Consequently, the researcher must decide whether to account for a theoretical endogeneity or a known design effect. The approach selected for this research ignores the possible endogeneity but accounts for sampling and design effects. The results, however, must be viewed with caution since it is not possible to disentangle utilization experience from perceptions of access or attitudinal barriers to care.

Measuring Volume of Physician Visits

In recent years, the most commonly used source of health services utilization data has consisted of response to surveys (Wolinsky, Mosley and Coe, 1986). The data collection technique for the Piedmont Health Survey of the Elderly also relies on subject recall. Consequently, the question of whether an elderly individual can or will respond accurately becomes important (Glandon, Counte and Tancredi, 1992). Systematic variance in reporting number of physician visits resulting in under-reporting (or over-reporting) will bias research findings even in large samples. Glandon, Counte and Tancredi (1992) analyzed the discrepancy between archival and self-report measures of physician utilization and examined the association of that discrepancy with health status and socio-demographic variables. Their findings indicate that lower health status is associated with over-reporting of utilization and higher levels of utilization are associated with under-reporting of physician visits. Apparently, the more visits an individual has the more difficult it is to recall the exact number of visits. For every visit increase as reported by the archival records, Glandon et al. found that the discrepancy increases by about .5 visits. However, relatively few subjects had difficulty recalling whether or not they had contact with a physician during the study period.

Consequences of using self-reported utilization data were demonstrated in the work of Cleary and Jette (1984). They estimated two models of utilization, one predicting self-reported utilization and the other archival utilization data from medical records. Comparing results from the two estimations, they found that coefficients significant in one equation were not necessarily significant in the second equation. More importantly, they found a systematic bias with under-reporting increasing with age of subject. There have been no comparable studies examining bias related to over- or under-reporting of delays in seeking medical care.

The implications of these findings for this research can be summarized by the following: 1) for the analysis that estimates the likelihood of any contact with a physician, recall bias is not a major threat (most subjects are able to recall if they had at least one visit with a physician); and 2) for the analysis that estimates the volume of physician visits these findings are problematic. One attempt to deal with the potential effect of the bias is to truncate the number of physician visits (visits equaling 12 or more are truncated to 12) thereby minimizing the recall bias. Another is to counsel the reader to examine the findings with caution, particularly any association between health status and utilization, as well as age and utilization.

EXTERNAL VALIDITY

According to Sechrest and Hannah (1990) external validity in non-experimental data refers to "the validity with which conclusions are drawn about the generalizability of relationships (correlational or causal) to and across populations of persons, settings, and times. The major issue is the researcher's tendency to extrapolate results to populations beyond those represented in the data (p. 2)." With this in mind, the main threat to external validity associated with this research concerns the generalizability of the results to care seeking behaviors and utilization of a physician by elderly people living in other regions. Although the sample is large, contains elderly subjects living in both metro and non-metro counties, and contains an over-sampling of African-American elderly, it is nonetheless, drawn from one region in the southern United States.

In addition, participants that required a proxy respondent are eliminated from this study. The need for proxy respondents increases with subject age and disability (Magaziner, 1992), therefore, it can be assumed that elders dropped from this study because of the need for proxy respondents are older and more frail than those respondents who were able to complete the interview. Consequently, generalizability of the findings from this study to frail, old-old, community residents must be made with caution.

NOTES

1. Landerman, L.R. (1992) Missing Value Imputations for EPESE Composites and Questionnaire Items. Piedmont Health Survey of the Elderly, Duke University. Draft.

2. For a discussion of adjustments for complex survey designs, see Kalton G., Introduction to Survey Sampling. Beverly Hills: Sage, 1983.

3. STATA Corporation, 702 University Drive East, College Station, TX 77840

4. SUDAAN: Professional Software for SUrvey DAta ANalysis. Research Triangle Park NC: Research Triangle Institute. 1989.

5. As the name implies, this method involves two successive applications of OLS. The process is as follows: Stage 1. To get rid of the likely correlation between Y_1 and u_2, Y_1 is regressed on all the predetermined variables in the whole system. A predicted Y_1 is obtained which is an estimate of the mean value of Y conditional upon the fixed X's not including the stochastic error term. Stage 2. Y_2 is then estimated including the predicted Y_1 rather than the actual value. As a result, OLS or logistic regression can be applied which will give consistent estimates of the parameters (Gujarati, 1988; p.604).

V

Findings

This chapter contains a presentation of the findings derived from the analysis of baseline data from the Piedmont Health Survey of the Elderly. The findings begin with descriptive statistics followed by a presentation of results from bivariate and multivariate analyses, which are arranged in two sections according to research questions related to delay of medical care and to utilization of physician visits. In addition, each section contains an examination of the role of race as potentially confounding or modifying relationships under study. The overall model underlying this research is presented in Chapter III and illustrated in Figure 3.1 According to this model, predisposing, enabling and need-for-care characteristics influence perceptions of access and/or attitudinal barriers to seeking medical care; in addition, these characteristics affect the use of physician visits directly as well as indirectly via their influence on perceived barriers. To facilitate the reader's navigation through the abundance of findings, each section is preceded by a component figure relevant to the aspect of the overall model under analysis. Furthermore, figures of direct and indirect effects are displayed in the last section of the chapter.

DESCRIPTIVE STATISTICS

The following section includes descriptive statistics for the independent (Table 5.1) and dependent variables (Table 5.2). All statistics are weighted and displayed for the combined sample as well as by race. Note that although the delay variables are included as dependent variables in Table 5.2, they are in fact outcome (or dependent) variables in the first phase of the analysis (examining characteristics associated with delay), and explanatory variables in the second phase of the analysis (examining physician visits).

Independent Variables

Predisposing Characteristics.   The following variables were used to measure predisposing characteristics: age, gender, race (black and white), marital status (married and not married), household composition (living alone and living with others) and education. As shown on Table 5.1, one-third of the weighted sample is composed of African-American elders. Mean age for the combined sample is 73, with a range of 65 to 101 years and a standard deviation of 6.3. It is the same for elderly blacks and elderly whites. Nearly 38 percent of the combined sample is male. This proportion does not vary by race. Approximately 52 percent of the total sample is married, however, there is nearly a 10 percent difference in marital status between black and white elders. Fifty-five percent of white elders are married as compared with 45 percent of black elders. This difference is statistically significant (p<.05).

Nearly 30 percent of the elders in this sample live alone. A slightly greater proportion of white elders live alone than do black elders (27 versus 31 percent). While this difference is not large, given the size of this sample, it is statistically significant. Years of schooling range from 0 to 17, with a mean of 9 years for the combined sample. Mean education level is higher for white elders as compared with black elders (10.3 versus 7.6). This difference is also statistically significant (p<.05).

Enabling Characteristics.   The following variables are included as enabling characteristics: income, insurance, usual source of care, social support and place of residence (rural versus non-rural). Overall, reported income is quite low. Twenty-nine percent of the combined sample report an annual income of less than 5,000 dollars a year; another 29 percent report an annual income ranging between 5,000 and 10,000 dollars; nearly 23 percent report an income ranging between 10,000 and 20,000 dollars annually; and, almost 20 percent report an annual income of 20,000 dollars or more. There are marked differences in income between elderly African-Americans and elderly whites living in this five-county region of North Carolina (see Table 5.1). Elderly blacks have a significantly lower income with nearly half reporting an annual income of less than 5,000 dollars, as compared with 19 percent of elderly whites who are comparably impoverished. At the other extreme, 27 percent of white elders report an income of 20,000 dollars or more as compared with only 5 percent of elderly blacks. This supports the work of Gibson and Jackson (1992) who found that African-American elderly are more likely to live in families with limited economic resources.

Table 5.1: Characteristics of the Sample: Weighted means and proportions for black elders, white elders and combined sample.

VARIABLE	Combined Sample (n=3,746) Mean (s.d.) or Percent	Black Elders (n=1,999) Mean (s.d.) or Percent	White Elders (n=1,747) Mean (s.d.) or Percent
Predisposing Characteristics			
Age (range 65–101)	73.03 (s.d. 6.3)	73.03 (s.d. 5.1)	73.02 (s.d. 7.4)
Race			
Black	34.4		
White	63.6		
Sex			
Male	37.9	37.8	38.0
Female	62.1	62.2	62.0
Marital Status[1]			
Married	51.8	45.1	55.3
Unmarried	48.2	54.9	44.7
Household Composition[2]			
Living Alone	29.9	27.4	31.3
Living with Others	70.1	72.7	68.7
Education (range 0–17)[3]	9.36 (s.d. 4.0)	7.55 (s.d. 3.3)	10.31 (s.d. 4.4)
Enabling Characteristics			
Income[1]			
$5,000	29.0	48.0	19.0
$5–9,999	28.9	31.9	27.3
$10–19,000	22.5	14.8	26.6
$20,000 +	19.6	5.3	27.1

Table 5.1 (continued)

VARIABLE	Combined Sample (n=3,746) Mean (s.d.) or Percent	Black Elders (n=1,999) Mean (s.d.) or Percent	White Elders (n=1,747) Mean (s.d.) or Percent
Insurance			
Medigap[1]	55.1	30.5	68.0
Medicaid[1]	5.2	9.1	3.2
HMO[2]	8.0	6.3	9.0
Usual Source of Care[1]			
Private Physician	78.2	59.8	87.8
Clinic or OPD	16.3	33.1	7.4
None	5.6	7.1	4.8
Social Support			
No relative to turn to	15.8	15.3	16.1
No friend to turn to[1]	11.9	14.5	10.6
No help when sick[4]	18.2	16.2	19.2
No help with transportation[1]	29.5	25.8	31.4
Rural Residence[1]	47.5	53.8	44.2
Need for Care Characteristics			
Self–rated Health[1]			
Excellent	15.4	12.1	17.1
Good	40.7	36.5	42.8
Fair	31.7	37.9	28.4
Poor	12.3	13.5	11.7
Illness Index			
Good	39.6	37.6	40.6
Fair	26.4	27.3	25.9
Poor	34.1	35.0	33.6
Any ADL Disability	15.5	16.6	15.0

1. Sig. tests comparing black and white elders p<.001.
2. Sig. tests comparing black and white elders p<.05.
3. Sig. tests comparing black and white elders p<.01.
4. Sig. tests comparing black and white elders p<.10.

Availability of insurance supplementary to Medicare was reported by 55 percent of the combined sample. This, too, varies considerably by race. Sixty-eight percent of white elders report having private health insurance supplementary to Medicare as compared with only 30 percent of elderly African-Americans. This is consistent with the work of Rice and McCall (1985) who found that white elders were more likely to purchase private insurance to supplement Medicare benefits as compared to black elders. While 5 percent of the combined sample are enrolled in Medicaid, a larger proportion of black elderly are recipients of Medicaid as compared with white elders (9.1 and 3.2 percent). This finding is compatible with the low income reported by black elders in the study.

Enrollment in a health maintenance organization is reported by only 8 percent of the sample (6 percent of blacks and 9 percent of whites). This is not surprising given the low penetration of health maintenance organizations in the health care market of this region at that time.

Black and white elders in this sample tend to receive their health care at different sites. Slightly more than 78 percent of the combined sample named a private physician as a usual source of care, however, examining source of care by race reveals that nearly 88 percent of white elders receive their care at a private physician's office as compared to 60 percent of blacks. In addition, 16 percent of the combined sample named a clinic as a source of care, however, stratification of this variable by race reveals that a third of black elders receive their health care from a clinic as compared to only 7 percent of white elders. A study conducted by Salber and colleagues (1976), which included parts of the Piedmont region encompassed in this study, found that the use of private physicians by blacks over the age of 65 ranged from 37 to 48 percent, while the use of clinics ranged from 48 to 56 percent. Comparable statistics for whites over age 65 were 73 to 85 percent being seen by a private physician and 10 to 17 percent being seen at a clinic. While exact comparisons between findings from the two studies cannot be made, these numbers suggest that the trend, for a greater proportion of elderly whites to be seen by a private physician, and for a larger proportion of elderly blacks to be seen at clinics, continues.

Overall, 5.6 percent of elders do not have a usual source of care. Stratification by race reveals that lack of a usual source of care is slightly more prevalent among black elders as compared with white elders (7 versus 5 percent). This finding is somewhat better than those among younger populations which report that African-Americans are almost twice as likely as whites to receive medical care in hospital clinics, emergency rooms, and other organized health care settings where the continuity of care is in doubt (Williams, 1992).

Nearly 16 percent of the combined sample lack at least one relative in whom the respondent could confide or could call on for assistance. This proportion is similar for blacks and whites. Lacking a friend for assistance or for serving as confidant, was reported by nearly 12 percent of the combined sample with proportions by race being nearly 15 percent for blacks and 11 percent for whites. Approximately 18 percent of elders received no assistance from another person for illness during the year prior to the interview. These proportions differ little by race (16 percent of blacks versus 19 percent of whites). Thirty percent of the combined sample did not receive assistance with transportation, with 26 percent of black elders and 31 percent of white elders receiving no assistance. It is not clear from the way the question was asked whether the subject needed help but did not receive it or whether no assistance was given because no help was requested or needed.

Approximately 48 percent of the elders in this five county region live in a rural county. A larger proportion of black elders live in one of the four rural counties as compared with white elders (54 versus 44 percent).

Need-for-Care Characteristics.   Variables measuring need-for-care include: self-rated health status, Illness Index and disability. Overall, 12 percent of elders view their health as poor, nearly 32 percent consider their health to be fair and 56 percent rate their health as good or excellent. A larger proportion of black elders rate their health as fair or poor compared with white elders (51 percent versus 40 percent). This finding is consistent with national data indicating that elderly blacks generally score lower than elderly whites on self-ratings of health status (National Center for Health Statistics, 1988).

The Illness Index is a measure of the presence and severity of disease. As measured by this index, nearly 40 percent of subjects are in good health, 26 percent in fair health and 34 percent in poor health. Despite racial differences in self-perceived health, these proportions are similar for both black and white elders. Disability, as measured by the inability to perform one or more tasks of daily living, is reported by nearly 16 percent of the combined sample; this proportion does not vary by race.

Dependent Variables

Delaying Medical Care. When asked whether they ever put off or postpone going to the doctor when they think they need to go, nearly 61 percent of the combined sample responded 'never', 27 percent responded 'occasionally', while 12 percent stated that they postpone or neglect going to the doctor 'often'. These proportions are quite similar for black and white elders (see Table 5.2).

Table 5.2: Characteristics of the Sample: Weighted Means and Percents for Outcome Variables.

VARIABLE	Combined Sample Mean (s.d.) or Percent	Black Elders Mean (s.d.) or Percent	White Elders Mean (s.d.) or Percent
Physician Visits			
Physician visits during the past year (n=3,476)			
NO visits during the past year	19.2	18.1	19.7
One or more visits	80.8	81.9	80.3
Number of visits AMONG USERS of care (n=3,016)	5.01 (s.d. 3.7) range 1– 12	5.10 (s.d. 3.6)	4.91 (s.d. 3.7)
Delaying Medical Care (n=3,746)			
Never	60.9	61.4	60.6
Occasionally	27.0	27.3	26.9
Often	12.1	11.3	12.5
Among Delayers: Reasons for Delaying Medical Care (n=1,468)			
Perceived Barriers to Access			
Concern with cost	51.7	53.6	49.6
Unsure where to go	11.8	13.0	10.6
Transportation or distance[1]	22.8	27.7	17.3
Attitudinal Barriers			
Going won't do any good[2]	29.4	22.5	36.9
Problem will get better by itself[2]	70.9	64.4	78.1

1. Significance tests comparing black and white elders p<.05.
2. Significance tests comparing black and white elders p<.01.

Among the 39 percent of elders who delayed medical care 'occasionally' or 'often', the most common reason given for delaying medical care is the belief that a problem would get better by itself (71 percent of the combined sample), followed by concern with cost as a reason for delay (nearly 52 percent). Twenty-nine percent stated that in the past year they did not go to the doctor because going would not do any good and nearly a fourth of the sample put off visiting a physician because of distance or transportation difficulties.

Reasons for delaying medical care differ by race. The proportion of elders who delay medical care because of perceived barriers to access (concern with cost, being unsure where to go for care and/or distance or transportation) is greater for blacks as compared with whites (these differences are statistically significant for distance or transportation only, but in the same direction for all three). On the other hand, the proportion of elders who delay medical care because of attitudinal barriers is greater for whites than for blacks. Nearly 78 percent of white elders who delay medical care do so because they believe problems will get better without intervention, as compared with 64 percent of blacks. Thirty-seven percent of white elderly delayers responded that they did so because they believe that going to the doctor would not do any good, compared with 23 percent of elderly blacks.

Reasons for Delay in Relation to Delaying Often. Table 5.3 displays the unadjusted odds ratios, among the 1,468 subjects who delay medical care, comparing occasional versus frequent reported delay.[1] Delaying because of concern with the cost of care more than doubles the odds of reporting frequent delay (2.36 for the combined sample). This finding is consistent among black and white elders. Uncertainty regarding where to seek medical care nearly doubles the odds of frequent delay among white elders and increases the odds among black elders by 35 percent (note that the confidence interval (CI) for the odds ratio (OR) for black elders contains unity and therefore is not deemed statistically significant). Black elders who delay because of distance or transportation difficulties increase their odds of frequent delay by nearly 60 percent while white elders who delay for this reason have a decrease in their odds of frequent delay (the 95% CI for the OR for whites contains unity). Attributing care seeking delay to doubts about the efficacy of a visit is associated with an 80 percent increase in the odds of frequent delay among black elders and a 60 percent increase in the odds of frequent delay among white elders. Although the belief that a problem will get better without medical intervention is the most common reason for delay, it is not associated with frequent delay.

Table 5.3: Among Delayers of Medical Care: Unadjusted Odds Ratios (OR) for Reasons for Delay, in Relationship to Delaying Often, by Race.*

Reason for Delay	Percent Delaying Often			Odds of Delaying Often			95% Confidence Interval		
	Black (N=769)	White (N=699)	Combined (N=1,468)	Black	White	Combined	Black	White	Combined
Perceived Barriers to Access									
Concern with cost	20.3	20.9	20.4	**2.36**	**2.31**	**2.34**	**(1.70, 3.27)**	**(1.68, 3.20)**	**(1.86, 2.94)**
Unsure where to go for care	4.6	5.1	4.8	1.35	**1.98**	**1.60**	(0.87, 2.10)	**(1.22, 3.21)**	**(1.16, 2.22)**
Difficulty with distance or transportation	10.1	5.3	7.8	**1.59**	0.89	1.25	**(1.14, 2.23)**	(0.58, 1.33)	(0.97, 1.63)
Attitudinal Barriers									
Going won't do any good	8.8	14.6	11.6	**1.80**	**1.60**	**1.68**	(1.26, 2.56)	**(1.1 6, 2.21)**	**(1.32, 2.13)**
Problem will get better by itself	19.4	24.3	21.7	1.10	0.70	0.91	(0.80, 1.10)	(0.48, 1.02)	(0.71, 1.16)

*OR's with 95% CI's that do not contain unity are deemed significant and are displayed in bold type.

In this study, delay is defined as postponing or *often* neglecting to seek care because of five reasons (concern with cost, unsure where to seek care, distance or transportation, going won't do any good and, the problem will resolve without intervention). The table below displays the proportion of subjects who delayed often, by reason and by race.

Although a larger proportion of elderly African-Americans than elderly whites give access barriers as reasons for *any* delay (see Table 5.2), the proportion of elderly blacks who delay *often* for these reasons is nearly the same as that of elderly whites (see Table 5.4). For example, 8 percent of the combined sample delay regularly because of concern with the cost of care; this proportion is the same for both blacks and whites. The only exception is a small racial difference for distance or transportation difficulties (4 percent of elderly blacks and 2 percent of elderly whites). However, a smaller proportion of elderly blacks delay often because of attitudinal barriers, as compared with elderly whites.

Table 5.4: Percent of Subjects Delaying Medical Care Often, by Reason and by Race.

Reason for Delay	Black Elders (N=1,999) %	White Elders (N=1,747) %	Combined Sample (N=3,746) %
Perceived Barriers to Access	8	8	8
Concern with Cost	8	8	8
Unsure where to go	2	2	2
Distance or transportation	4	2	3
Attitudinal Barriers			
Going won't do any good	3	6	5
Problem will get better by itself	7	10	9

Physician Visits

Two indicators of physician visits are included as outcome variables; these are a measure of *contact* (no visit during the year preceding the interview versus one or more visits) and a measure of *volume* (number of visits among those with one or more visits). Nineteen percent of elders in the study had no annual contact with a physician during the year preceding the interview (see Table 5.2). This proportion is similar for black and white elders (18 percent of the former and nearly 20 percent of the latter). Among those with at least one physician visit, the average number of physician visits during a 12 month period is 5. The average number of visits is essentially the same for black and white elders.

ANALYSIS OF THE DETERMINANTS OF DELAY

Research Question: Who delays seeking needed medical care, and why?

Figure 5.1: Predisposing, Enabling and Need-for-Care Characteristics and Delay

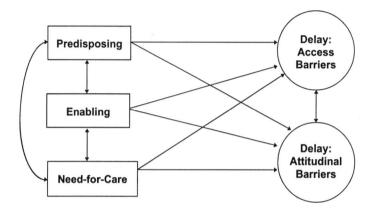

As indicated by Figure 5.1, the findings presented in this section result from an analysis of subject characteristics in relation to delay in seeking medical care attributed to access and/or attitudinal barriers. This section partially addresses another research question namely, the role of race in the relationship of subject characteristics and the five measures of delay. In this analysis, delay is defined as postponing or *often* neglecting to seek care because of five reasons (concern with cost, unsure where to seek care, distance or transportation, going won't do any good and, the problem will resolve without intervention). The reasons for delay are not mutually exclusive categories; a subject could attribute delay to as many reasons as apply. Consequently, five analyses were conducted; each reason for delay was analyzed as a separate outcome variable. This section begins with the results of the bivariate analysis between subject characteristic and each outcome followed by results of multivariate modeling.

Bivariate Analysis.

Tables 5.5 and 5.6 display weighted unadjusted odds ratios for the predisposing, enabling and need-for-care characteristics in relation to each of the delay variables. Odds ratios whose 95% confidence intervals do not contain unity are deemed significant and are highlighted in bold lettering. The results are displayed in two sections: one examines characteristics associated with delay attributed to perceived barriers to access, the second examines characteristics associated with delay attributed to attitudinal barriers.

Delaying Medical Care Because of Perceived Barriers to Access

The results of bivariate analysis of predisposing, enabling and need-for-care characteristics in relation to the three access reasons for delay (cost, uncertainty regarding location and distance or transportation) are given below (see Table 5.5).

Predisposing Characteristics. These characteristics include age, gender, race, marital status, living alone and years of education. Several significant findings emerge in this bivariate analysis. Looking across the three outcome variables, age, race, marital status and education are associated with delay. As age increases the odds of delaying medical care because of concern with the cost of care decrease; the odds displayed compare age 65 with age 75. Age, however, is not associated with any other reason for delay. Being an elderly black nearly doubles the odds of delaying medical care because of distance or transportation difficulties: the odds for elderly blacks is 1.98, as compared with elderly whites. Married elders are less likely to delay medical care because of distance or transportation difficulties, as compared with non-married elders (OR = .51) and, as education increases, the odds of delaying medical care because of perceived access decreases. The odds ratio for 12 years of education, as compared with 6 years of education, is .52 for concern with the cost of care and .32 for distance or transportation difficulties.

Enabling Characteristics. Not surprisingly, as income increases the odds of delaying because of concern with cost and because of distance or transportation difficulties decrease. This trend also holds for delays attributed to uncertainty about where to seek care, however, the confidence interval is wide and contains unity. Reporting a clinic as the site of medical care does not alter the odds of delaying often because of concern with cost or knowing where to go, it is, however, associated with a 90 percent increase in the odds of delay attributed to distance or transportation problems. Since a greater proportion of those seeking care in clinics are black elders, and black elders are more likely to delay for this reason, race may very well interact with or confound the relationship between receiving care at a clinic and delaying for this reason. Lacking a usual source of care is associated with an increase in the odds of delaying

Table 5.5: Weighted Unadjusted Odds Ratios (OR) and Confidence Intervals by Subject Characteristics in Relation to Delaying Medical Care Because of Perceived Access Barriers.*

Subject Characteristics	Concern With Cost OR (95% CI)	Don't Know Where to Go for Care OR (95% CI)	Distance or Transportation Difficulties OR (95% CI)
Predisposing			
Age[a]	0.66 (0.51, 0.87)	0.90 (0.51, 1.59)	1.25 (0.92, 1.69)
Gender (Male=1)	0.86 (0.62, 1.18)	0.76 (0.39, 1.45)	0.61 (0.34, 1.07)
Race (Black=1)	0.96 (0.73, 1.27)	0.86 (0.49, 1.48)	**1.98 (1.28, 3.08)**
Marital Status (Married=1)	1.06 (0.81, 1.38)	1.00 (0.60, 1.68)	**0.51 (0.31, .83)**
Living Alone (Alone=1)	0.89 (0.67, 1.18)	1.02 (0.59, 1.76)	1.29 (0.82, 2.02)
Years of Education[b]	**0.52 (0.41, 0.65)**	0.68 (0.42, 1.09)	**0.32 (0.24, 0.44)**
Enabling			
Income			
$5,000[c]			
$5–9,999	0.88 (0.66, 1.17)	1.02 (0.56, 1.86)	**0.59 (0.36, 0.97)**
$10–19,999	**0.41 (0.25, 0.65)**	0.66 (0.29, 1.48)	**0.26 (0.11, 0.61)**
$20,000 +	**0.23 (0.12, 0.44)**	0.59 (0.21, 1.73)	**0.02 (0.00, 0.17)**
Usual Source of Care			
Private physician office [c]			
Clinic	1.20 (0.84, 1.72)	0.94 (0.49, 1.80)	**1.90 (1.15, 3.14)**
No usual source	1.50 (0.92, 2.44)	**2.76 (1.33, 5.72)**	**2.59 (1.17, 5.74)**
Insurance			
Medigap	**0.52 (0.38, 0.70)**	0.98 (0.55, 1.75)	**0.38 (0.24, 0.61)**
Medicaid	1.10 (0.68, 1.79)	1.78 (0.82, 3.88)	**2.40 (1.27, 4.55)**
Health maintenance org.	0.86 (0.47, 1.58)	1.36 (0.38, 4.85)	0.31 (0.09, 1.04)
Social Support			
No relatives to turn to	**1.65 (1.16, 2.34)**	**2.25 (1.18, 4.28)**	1.58 (0.92, 2.72)
No friends to turn to	0.82 (0.54, 1.25)	0.85 (0.42, 1.70)	0.93 (0.54, 1.59)
No assistance for illness	**0.61 (0.40, 0.91)**	0.62 (0.27, 1.41)	0.77 (0.43, 1.39)
No assistance with transportation	0.77 (0.57, 1.05)	0.74 (0.40, 1.38)	**0.52 (0.32, 0.86)**

Table 5.5 (continued)

Subject Characteristics	Concern With Cost OR (95% CI)	Don't Know Where to Go for Care OR (95% CI)	Distance or Transportation Difficulties OR (95% CI)
Rural Residence (yes=1),	1.64 (1.20, 2.23),	1.18 (0.66, 2.11)	1.30 (0.82, 2.04)
Need for Care			
Self-perceived health status			
excellent/good [c]			
fair	**2.70 (1.94, 3.75)**	**2.81 (1.30, 6.09)**	**2.45 (1.39, 4.32)**
poor	**6.61 (4.68, 9.32)**	**4.08 (1.82, 9.15)**	**7.32 (4.18, 12.82)**
Illness Index			
good health [c]			
fair health	1.06 (0.75, 1.49)	0.75 (0.36, 1.57)	1.34 (0.76, 2.36)
poor health	1.06 (0.76, 1.46)	0.69 (0.35, 1.36)	0.82 (0.49, 1.37)
Functional Disability (Any=1)	**1.45 (1.01, 2.08)**	1.31 (0.65, 2.63)	**1.89 (1.09, 3.28)**

* OR whose 95% CI does not contain unity is displayed in bold type.

a – odds ratio compares a 65 year old to a 75 year old

b – odds ratio compares 6 years of education with 12 years

c – reference category

medical care because of all three access reasons. For example, elders who lack a usual source of medical care are nearly three times more likely to neglect to seek care often because of uncertainty as to where to seek care (OR 2.76), as compared with elders who name a private physician office as a regular source of care.

The effect of having insurance in addition to Medicare is mixed. The availability of Medigap insurance is associated with a significant decrease in the odds of delaying because of cost (OR .52) and transportation difficulties (OR .38) but does not alter the odds of delaying because of not knowing where to seek help (OR .98). Medicaid insurance is associated with an increase in delaying because of transportation difficulties (OR 2.40) and not knowing where to go for help (OR 1.78, 95% CI .82, 3.88) but is not associated with delaying because of concern with cost (OR 1.10). Belonging to a health maintenance organization does not have a statistically significant association with delaying medical care.

The effect of social support is puzzling. Lacking relatives to serve as confidants or to ask for assistance is associated with an increase in the odds of delaying needed medical care because of perceived barriers to access (with the exception of distance or transportation which is in a positive direction, although the confidence interval contains unity). However, lacking friends has no statistically significant effect on delay. Instrumental support (receiving assistance for illness or transportation) has a more consistent effect: elders who did not receive assistance from another individual for illness and elders who were not assisted with transportation were found to have a decrease in the odds of often delaying medical care because of perceived barriers to access (see Table 5.5). Surprisingly, elders who did *not* receive assistance with transportation were also *less* likely to attribute delay to distance or transportation difficulties (OR .52), leaving open the possibility that those who did not receive assistance with transportation were not in need of any.

Living in a rural county is associated with an increase in the odds of delaying medical care because of concern with cost (OR = 1.64), but no statistically significant association with the other two measures of perceived barriers to access.

Need-for-Care Characteristics. Poor self-ratings of health, as compared with ratings of excellent or good, is associated with a striking increase in the odds of neglecting to seek care because of concern with cost (6.61), not knowing where to go for care (4.08), and distance or transportation difficulties (7.32). Paradoxically, the presence of illness, as

Table 5.6: Weighted Unadjusted Odds Ratios (OR) for Subject Characteristic in Relation to Delaying Medical Care Because of Attitudinal Barriers.*

Characteristic (n=3,746)	Going to the Doctor Will Not Do Any Good OR (95% CI)	Problem Will Get Better By Itself OR (95% CI)
Predisposing		
Age[a]	0.97 (0.71, 1.33)	0.84 (0.55, 1.28)
Gender (Male=1)	1.25 (0.86, 1.83)	0.84 (0.64, 1.13)
Race (Black=1)	**0.55 (0.39, 0.77)**	**0.75 (0.57, 0.98)**
Marital Status (Married=1)	**1.41 (1.01, 1.98)**	1.14 (0.89, 1.46)
Living Alone (Alone=1)	0.76 (0.54, 1.08)	0.92 (0.71, 1.19)
Years of Education[b]	**0.72 (0.68, 0.75)**	**0.70 (0.67, 0.72)**
Enabling		
Income		
$5,000[c]		
$5–9,999	1.28 (0.88, 1.89)	0.95 (0.70, 1.29)
$10– 19,999	0.84 (0.49, 1.44)	0.71 (0.48, 1.07)
$20,000 +	0.71 (0.40, 1.28)	**0.52 (0.32, 0.83)**
Usual Source of Care		
Private physician office[c]		
Clinic	1.11 (0.66, 1.86)	1.29 (0.88, 1.88)
No usual source	**2.36 (1.36, 4.09)**	**1.65 (1.03, 2.64)**
Insurance		
Medigap	0.82 (0.56, 1.21)	0.79 (0.61, 1.01)
Medicaid	0.78 (0.40, 1.52)	1.34 (0.84, 2.12)
HMO	0.94 (0.41, 2.14)	0.99 (0.58, 1.67)
Social Support		
No relatives to turn to	**1.91 (1.24, 2.94)**	**1.46 (1.02, 2.08)**
No friends to turn to	0.77 (0.47, 1.28)	0.68 (0.45, 1.04)
No assistance when ill	0.91 (0.55, 1.52)	0.69 (0.47, 1.02)
No assistance with transportation	1.00 (0.69, 1.45)	0.90 (0.68, 1.19)
Rural Residence (yes=1)	1.19 (0.81, 1.74)	**1.75 (1.31, 2.33)**
Need–for–Care		
Self–perceived health status excellent/good[c]		
fair	**1.95 (1.26, 3.01)**	**1.76 (1.27, 2.46)**
poor	**3.24 (2.10, 5.01)**	**2.51 (1.76, 3.60)**
Illness Index good health[c]		
fair health	0.88 (0.53, 1.46)	0.91 (0.65, 1.28)
poor health	1.04 (0.68, 1.59)	0.79 (0.56, 1.12)
Disability (Any=1)	**1.55 (1.01, 2.36)**	1.14 (0.76, 1.71)

* OR whose 95% Confidence Interval (95% CI) does not contain
 unity is displayed in bold type.
a – odds ratio compares a 65 year old to a 75 year old
b – odds ratio compares 6 years of education with 12 years
c – reference category

measured by the Illness Index, does not have a statistically significant association with delaying medical care (see Table 5.5). Lastly, the presence of functional disability behaves more like self-rated health than the Illness Index, albeit not as strong, in its association with delay (OR for cost = 1.45; OR for transportation = 1.89).

Delaying Medical Care Often Because of Attitudinal Barriers

This section includes the results of the bivariate analysis of the relationship between predisposing, enabling and need-for-care characteristics and delaying medical care because of attitudinal reasons (going would not do any good and problems would get better by themselves). The findings are displayed in Table 5.6.

Predisposing Characteristics. Black elders are less likely to delay medical care because of attitudinal barriers as compared with white elders (OR = .55 for delaying because of the belief that going would not do any good and an OR = .75 for delaying often because of the belief that a problem would get better by itself). Education is also associated with a lowering of the odds of regularly delaying for these reasons; the OR for 12 years of education is .72 that of 6 years of education. Married elders are more likely to delay medical care because of believing that a visit would not do any good than unmarried persons (OR 1.41). The confidence intervals for the odds ratios for age, gender and living alone in relation to regularly delaying medical care for these reasons contain unity (see Table 5.6).

Enabling Characteristics. There is a trend for the odds ratio for both outcomes to decrease as income increases. The only significant finding, however, is that for the highest income category. The odds of an individual whose annual income exceeds 20,000 dollars delaying often because of the belief that medical problems will get better without intervention is approximately half that of one whose income is less than 5,000 dollars a year.

Comparing elders who receive their care at a private physician's office with elders who receive their care at a clinic reveals no substantive differences in the odds of delaying for attitudinal reasons, however, having *no* usual source of care is associated with an increase in the odds of delaying medical care often because of attitudinal barriers (OR of 2.36 and 1.65).

Medigap insurance, Medicaid insurance or participation in a health maintenance organization are not associated with attributing delays in seeking medical care to attitudinal barriers.

Once again, the effect of the social support measures are mixed and somewhat puzzling. Lacking relatives to turn to is associated with an increase in the odds of delaying because of attitudinal barriers. This attribute is associated with nearly doubling the odds of attributing delay in seeking needed medical care to doubts about the potential efficacy of a visit (OR 1.91), as well as increase the odds of delaying because of the belief symptoms would resolve on their own (OR 1.46). On the other hand, lack of friends for confidences or assistance is associated with a *decrease* in the odds of delaying because of believing the problem to be self-limiting (OR = .68) and with the odds of believing that going to a doctor would not do any good (OR = .77), note, however, that the 95 percent confidence intervals for these two odds ratios contain unity. Elders who did not receive assistance with illness were less likely to believe that a problem would get better without intervention (OR = .69) while no assistance with transportation is not associated with delay for attitudinal reasons.

Elders living in a rural county are more likely than their non-rural counterparts to delay because they believe the problem to be self-limiting, as compared with elders living in a non-rural county (OR 1.75). However, rural residence does not have a significant association with the belief that going to the doctor would not do any good (OR 1.19).

Need-for-Care Characteristics. Among the need-for-care variables, self-rated health is strongly associated with delaying because of attitudinal barriers; particularly for elderly subjects who rate their health as poor (OR 3.24 and 2.51). Interestingly, the Illness Index is associated with delaying for these reasons while the presence of disability (as measured by the Katz scale) increases the odds of delaying because of believing the visit would not do any good (OR 1.55) but not because of believing that the problem would get better by itself.

Summary of the Bivariate Analysis of Subject Characteristics and Delay

Table 5.7 displays a summary of the direction of effect between predisposing, enabling and need-for-care characteristics and delay. Rather than displaying odds ratios and confidence intervals, symbols are used: 1) a plus sign indicates an increase in the odds, 2) a minus sign indicates a decrease in the odds and, 3) a blank space indicates no association (an odds ratio whose 95 percent confidence interval contains unity).

Table 5.7: Summary of Bivariate Analysis: Increase (+) or Decrease (−) in the Odds of Regularly Delaying Medical Care in Relation to Predisposing, Enabling and Need–for–Care Characteristics.*

VARIABLES	Concern with Cost	Unsure Where to go	Distance or Transportation	Going Won't do any Good	Get Better by Itself
Predisposing					
Age	−				
Gender (Male=1)					
Race (Black=1)			+	−	−
Married (yes=1)			−		
Living alone (yes=1)					
Education	−		−	−	−
Enabling					
Income	−		−		−
Insurance					−
Medigap	−	+	−		
Medicaid		+	+		
HMO			−		
Usual Source of Care					
Clinic			+		
None	+	+	+	+	+
Social Support					
No relative to turn to	+	+	+	+	+
No friend to turn to					
No help when sick	−				
No help with transportation			−		
Rural Residence	+				+
Need for Care					
Self Perceived Health	+	+	+	+	+
Illness Index	+			+	
Any Disability (yes=1)	+		+	+	

*Note: biavariable results which revealed no change in the odds are left blank.

Looking across the five outcome variables a number of patterns emerge. Increased income and education are consistently associated with a decrease in the odds of delay, while lacking a usual source of care, lack of relatives and fair or poor self-ratings of health are characteristics associated with an increase in the odds of delay across the five reasons. On the other hand, gender, household composition (living alone) and the Illness Index have no significant association with delay.

Research Question: Does race mediate delay in seeking medical care?

Unadjusted and Adjusted Odds Ratios for Race in Relation to Delaying Because of Perceived Access

Prior to estimating multivariate models of the delay outcomes, each variable is examined as a potential confounder or effect modifier of the relationship between race and the outcomes. Table 5.8 displays the unadjusted and adjusted (one variable at a time) odds ratios and 95 percent confidence intervals for race in relation to regularly delaying medical care because of perceived barriers to access. Findings highlighted in bold lettering indicate that the characteristic confounds the relationship between race and the outcome[2]; while starred findings indicate that the characteristic modifies the relationship between race and the outcome (these interactions are explored more thoroughly in the multivariate analysis).

Among the predisposing characteristics, education is the only variable which confounds the relationship between race and delay attributed to concern with the cost of care. The unadjusted odds ratio indicates that black elders are no more likely to delay for this reason than white elders (OR = .96, 95% CI .73, 1.26); however, adjusting for education reveals an odds ratio for black elders which is only .67 that of white elders (95% CI .49, .90). Education also confounds the relationship between race and delay attributed to uncertainty about where to seek care; the OR for black elders drops from .86 to .68 after adjusting for education, however, the confidence interval still contains unity. Finally, education modifies the relationship between race and delay because of distance or transportation difficulties, as does age. Both these variables will be included in the multivariate estimation along with the interaction terms.

In the unadjusted analysis, race has a negative, although weak, association with delay because uncertainty about where to seek care (OR .86, 95% CI .49, 1.48). Adjusting for education, income and self-per-

Table 5.8: Race and delaying medical care because of perceived barriers to access: Unadjusted and adjusted odds ratios (OR) and confidence intervals (CI).*

	Concern with Cost of Care OR (95% CI)	Unsure Where to Go for Care OR (95% CI)	Distance or Transportation OR (95% CI)
OR for Race, Unadjusted	0.96 (0.73, 1.26)	0.86 (0.49, 1.48)	1.98 (1.28, 3.08)
OR for Race, Adjusted for:			
Predisposing Characteristics:			
Age	0.96 (0.73, 1.26)	0.86 (0.49, 1.48)	**
Gender (Male=1)	0.96 (0.73, 1.26)	0.86 (0.49, 1.48)	1.98 (1.28, 3.08)
Married (yes=1)	0.96 (0.73, 1.27)	0.86 (0.50, 1.47)	1.87 (1.20, 2.89)
Living alone (yes=1)	0.95 (0.72, 1.26)	0.86 (0.49, 1.49)	2.01 (1.29, 3.11)
Education	**0.67 (0.49, 0.90)**	**0.68 (0.39, 1.18)**	**
Enabling Characteristics:			
Income	**0.65 (0.49, 0.88)**	**0.71 (0.41, 1.21)**	**1.20 (0.76, 1.90)**
Insurance			
Medigap	**0.72 (0.53, 0.98)**	0.83 (0.47, 1.46)	**1.48 (0.92, 2.39)**
Medicaid	0.95 (0.72, 1.26)	0.82 (0.47, 1.41)	**1.88 (1.18, 2.97)**
HMO	0.96 (0.72, 1.26)	0.86 (0.50, 1.49)	**1.94 (1.25, 3.03)**
Usual Source of Care	**	0.82 (0.46, 1.46)	**1.73 (1.06, 2.83)**
Social Support			
No relative to turn to	0.96 (0.73, 1.27)	0.86 (0.50, 1.49)	**1.99 (1.28, 3.09)**
No friend to turn to	0.96 (0.73, 1.27)	0.86 (0.50, 1.49)	**1.99 (1.28, 3.09)**
No help when sick	0.95 (0.72, 1.25)	0.84 (0.49, 1.47)	**1.97 (1.29, 3.06)**
No help with transportation	0.94 (0.72, 1.25)	0.84 (0.48, 1.47)	**
Rural Residence	**	0.84 (0.49, 1.46)	**1.94 (1.25, 3.00)**
Need–for–Care Characteristics:			
Self Perceived Health	**	**0.76 (0.44, 1.31)**	**1.80 (1.15, 2.82)**
Illness Index	**0.96 (0.72, 1.26)**	0.86 (0.50, 1.50)	1.98 (1.28, 3.07)
Any Disability (yes=1)	**0.95 (0.72, 1.26)**	0.85 (0.49, 1.48)	1.96 (1.26, 3.05)

* – numbers in bold highlight results which confound the relationship between race and the outcome.
** – interaction statistically significant (at the $p<.05$ level or below), therefore adjusted OR is irrelevant.

ceived health (one confounder at a time) alters the OR somewhat, however, the confidence interval still contains unity. No interactions with race were found to be statistically significant.

The unadjusted odds of elderly blacks regularly delaying medical care because of distance or transportation difficulties is nearly twice that of white elders (OR 1.98, 95% CI 1.28, 3.08). This finding is substantively altered by income and the availability of Medigap insurance; these two variables confound the relationship between race and delays attributed to this reason. After adjusting for income the OR decreases to 1.2 and the 95% confidence interval now contains unity (.76, 1.90); adjusting for supplementary insurance to Medicare results in an odds ratio of 1.48 and again, the 95% confident interval contains unity (.92, 2.39). Adjusting for usual source of care reveals that this variable is a weak confounder of the relationship between race and delay attributed to this reason (OR drops to 1.73, 95% CI 1.06, 2.83).

Education and *not* receiving assistance with transportation were found to modify the relationship between race and delays in medical care attributed to distance or transportation difficulties (the interaction term was statistically significant at p<.05). These two variables, as well as their interaction terms, were included, along with race, in the multivariate models and discussed later in this chapter.

Unadjusted and Adjusted Odds Ratios for Race in Relation to Delaying Because of Attitudinal Barriers

Unadjusted and adjusted odds ratios, and 95% confidence intervals, for race in relation to regularly delaying medical care because of attitudinal barriers are displayed in Table 5.9. The unadjusted odds ratios reveal that the proportion of black elders who regularly delay medical care because of attitudinal barriers is lower than that of white elders (OR .55 and .75). Among the predisposing variables, education is the only characteristic that confounds the association between race and attitudinal barriers. Adjusting for education results in a decrease in the odds ratio for black elders in relation to the belief that going to a doctor would not do any good, from .55 to .42 that of white elders; while the odds ratio in relation to the belief that problems would resolve without intervention decreases from .75 to .59 that of white elders. Adjusting for income results in a similar effect.

Table 5.9: Race and delaying medical care because of perceived
barriers to access: Unadjusted and adjusted odds ratios (OR)
and confidence intervals.*

	Going to the Doctor Will Not Do Any Good OR (95% CI)	Problem Will Get Better By Itself OR (95% CI)
OR for Race, Unadjusted	0.55 (0.39, 0.77)	0.75 (0.57, 0.98)
OR for Race, Adjusted for:		
Predisposing Characteristics:		
Age	0.54 (0.38, 0.77)	0.75 (0.57, 0.98)
Gender (Male=1)	0.55 (0.39, 0.77)	0.75 (0.57, 0.98)
Married (yes=1)	0.56 (0.40, 0.80)	0.76 (0.58, 1.00)
Living alone (yes=1)	0.54 (0.38, 0.77)	0.75 (0.57, 0.98)
Education	**0.42 (0.29, 0.62)**	**0.59 (0.45, 0.79)**
Enabling Characteristics:		
Income	**0.46 (0.32, 0.66)**	**0.60 (0.45, 0.80)**
Insurance		
Medigap	**0.47 (0.32, 0.68)**	0.79 (0.61, 1.01)
Medicaid	0.55 (0.39, 0.77)	0.73 (0.55, 0.97)
HMO	0.55 (0.38, 0.77)	0.75 (0.57, 0.98)
Usual Source of Care	**	**
Social Support		
No relative to turn to	0.55 (0.39, 0.78)	0.75 (0.57, 0.99)
No friend to turn to	0.55 (0.39, 0.78)	0.76 (0.58, 1.00)
No help when sick	0.55 (0.38, 0.77)	0.74 (0.56, 0.97)
No help with transportation	0.55 (0.39, 0.77)	0.74 (0.56, 0.98)
Rural Residence	0.54 (0.38, 0.76)	0.71 (0.54, 0.92)
Need for Care Characteristics:		
Self Perceived Health	0.50 (0.35, 0.70)	**
Illness Index	0.55 (0.39, 0.77)	0.75 (0.57, 0.99)
Any Disability (yes=1)	0.54 (0.38, 0.77)	0.75 (0.57, 0.98)

* – numbers in bold highlight results which confound the relationship
between race and the outcome.

** – interaction is statistically significant (at the $p<.05$ or below),
therefore, adjusted OR is irrelevant.

Adjusting for the availability of health insurance in addition to Medicare reveals that supplementary insurance to Medicare (Medigap) is a weak confounder of one of the outcomes (OR for the "going to the doctor would not do any good" outcome decreases to .47 from .55). Having a usual source of medical care modifies the relationship between race and both outcomes, while self-rated health modifies the relationship between race and the belief that problems would get better by themselves. The remaining characteristics neither confound nor modify the relationship between race and delay attributed to attitudinal barriers.

Multivariate Analysis of Delay in Seeking Medical Care

Five multivariate logistic models were estimated, and odds ratios and 95 percent confidence intervals calculated approximating the relative risk of reporting frequent delay for older adults in a particular group. Initially, for each of the five outcome variables, a full model was estimated that included all the predisposing, enabling and need-for-care characteristics. Then, attempts at paring down each model included the removal of variables that were non-significant in the bivariate analysis (see summary Table 5.7). In addition, all variables that were found to modify the association between race and the outcome variables were included as interaction terms and evaluated in the multivariate analysis (see Tables 5.8 and 5.9). Models were then re-estimated, the coefficients of the remaining variables examined and log-likelihood ratio tests conducted. These steps were repeated until a final model was obtained. The results of modeling are shown on Tables 5.10 and 5.11. Note that variables that do include an estimate for a particular outcome were evaluated, found not to have a meaningful association with the outcomes and, consequently, were not included in the reported model. Reported models were estimated using the SUDAAN software, which properly incorporates all relevant features of this complex sample design (i.e., PSU, stratification, cluster sampling and sample weights).

The multivariate findings are presented in two sections. The first presents the three measures of delay attributed to perceived barriers to access (concern with cost, unsure where to go for care and distance or transportation difficulties) while the second presents the two measures of delay attributed to attitudinal barriers (believing a visit would not do any good and believing problems would resolve without intervention).

Table 5.10 : Multivariate Analysis: Predisposing, Enabling and Need–for–Care Characteristics in Relation to Regularly Delaying Medical Care Because of Perceived Barriers to Access.

Characteristic (n=3,746)	Concern with Cost OR (95% CI)	Unsure Where to Go for Care OR (95% CI)	Distance or Transportation OR (95% CI)
Predisposing Characteristics			
Age[a]	0.55 (0.46, 0.71)		
Race (Black=1)	see below		
Gender (Male=1)			
Marital Status (Married=1)	**1.42 (1.00, 2.00)**		
Living Alone			
Education[b]	0.73 (0.54, 0.98)		0.57 (0.36, 0.89)
Enabling Characteristics			
Income			
$5,000[c]			
$5–9,999	0.84 (0.60, 1.20)		0.76 (0.45, 1.30)
$10– 19,999	**0.38 (0.22, 0.64)**		0.48 (0.19, 1.24)
$20,000 +	**0.25 (0.40, 0.56)**		**0.07 (0.01, 0.51)**
Insurance			
Medicare only[c]			
Medigap			
Medicaid			
HMO			
Usual Source of Care			
Private[c]			
Other (OPD, Clinic)	1.12 (0.78, 1.60)	0.85 (0.44, 1.64)	1.33 (0.80, 2.23)
None	**1.75 (0.98, 3.12)**	**2.80 (1.26, 6.24)**	**2.60 (1.15, 3.61)**
Social Support			
No relative to turn to		**2.08 (1.00, 4.32)**	
No friend to turn to			
No assistance when sick			
No assistance with transportation			
Rural Residence			
	see below		
Need for Care Characteristics			
Self Perceived Health			
Excel./good[c]			
Fair	**2.31 (1.68, 3.17)**	**3.24 (1.68, 6.26)**	**2.04 (1.15,3.61)**
Poor	**5.29 (3.66, 7.68)**	**5.11 (2.29, 11.37)**	**5.64 (3.12, 10.21)**
Illness Index			
Good health[c]			
Fair health	0.91 (0.65, 1.29)	0.68 (0.74, 1.36)	1.22 (0.70, 2.14)
Poor health	**0.66 (0.47, 0.93)**	0.50 (0.25, 1.01)	**0.53 (0.31, 0.92)**
Any disability (Yes=1)			
Interaction with Race			
Race and Rural Residence:			
Rural Black Elders	**0.68 (0.46, 0.92)**		
Non–rural Black Elders	**0.34 (0.21, 0.56)**		
Rural White Elders	0.97 (0.67, 1.41)		
Non–rural White Elders[c]	1.00		

a – odds ratio compares age 65 with age 75.

b – odds ratio compares 6 with 12 years of education.

c – reference category.

Delays in Seeking Medical Care Attributed to Access Barriers

Table 5.10 displays the adjusted odds ratios and 95 percent confidence intervals for predisposing, enabling and need-for-care characteristics in relation to attributing delays in seeking medical to access barriers.

Predisposing Characteristics. Six predisposing characteristics were evaluated: age, race, gender, marital status, living alone and education. Four predisposing characteristics, age, race, marital status and education, were included in the final model estimating the likelihood of attributing delay to cost concerns. As with the bivariate findings, increasing age is associated with a decreasing odds of regularly neglecting to seek care for this reason (OR for an individual aged 75 is .55 that of a 65 year old). In the cost equation, the interaction between race and rural residence is statistically significant. Surprisingly, being married results in a 42 percent increase in the odds of delaying often because of concern with cost. And, as years of education increase, the odds of delaying for this reason decrease (OR for 12 years of education is .73 that of 6 years of education).

In the bivariate analysis (see Table 5.5) race, marital status and education were associated with delay because of distance or transportation difficulties. In addition, adjusting for race revealed an interaction between race and education and race and age (see Table 5.8). However, in the multivariate modeling the only predisposing characteristic remaining in the equation is education, both interaction terms were no longer statistically significant and were removed from the model. As years of education increase, the odds of delaying often because of distance or transportation difficulties decrease; the odds for 12 years of education are .57 that of 6 years of education (see Table 5.10). Despite the strong association between race and delay because of distance or transportation difficulties in the bivariate analysis, in the multivariate model (adjusting for income and education), race was no longer a determinant of delay for this reason. None of the predisposing characteristics were included in the final model of delay attributed to uncertainty about where to seek medical care.

Enabling Characteristics. Five enabling characteristics were evaluated: income, insurance usual source of care, social support and rural residence. Looking across the three models estimated, some patterns emerge. For two of the three outcomes, concern with cost and distance or transportation difficulties, increased income is associated with a decrease in the odds of delaying medical care. This is particularly so for elders whose annual income is 20,000 dollars or more; the odds of an elder in this highest income category delaying medical care because of concern with cost is .25 that of an elder with an annual income less than 5,000 dollars, while the odds of delaying because of distance or transportation difficulties is only .07. Clearly, income is strongly associated with the elderly person's perception of access (see Table 5.10). Interestingly, income is not associated with uncertainty about where to seek care.

Compared with elders who report a private physician office as their usual source of care, elders without a regular source of care are more likely to delay medical care because of concern with cost (OR 1.75), uncertainty about where to seek care (2.80) and distance or transportation difficulties (OR 2.60). However, reporting a clinic as a usual source of care does not significantly alter the odds of delaying medical care for reasons of access.

Surprisingly, lack of network (friends or family), or instrumental social support (assistance with illness or transportation), does not alter perceptions of access to Medical Care. There is one exception, elders who have no relatives to rely on, or confide in, more than double their odds of delaying often because of uncertainty about where to seek care (OR 2.08, 95% CI 1.00, 4.32).

Need-for-Care Characteristics. These characteristics include three measures of health status: self-rated health, Illness Index and the presence of disability. As with the bivariate analysis, in the multivariate model self-ratings of health continue to play an important role in the perceptions of access to care. The odds of delaying for these reasons increase as self-ratings of health worsen; for example, compared with excellent or good rating of health, poor rating of health is associated with greater than a five-fold increase in the odds of delaying medical care because of concern with cost (OR 5.29), uncertainty about where to seek care (5.11) and distance or transportation difficulties (5.64). On the other hand, the presence and severity of medical illness (Illness Index) is associated with a decrease in the odds of delaying for these reasons, so that, as the severity of illness increases the odds of delay decrease; for example, elders who are in poor health, as measured by the Illness Index, have an odds of .50 that of elders who are in good health of delaying medical care often because of being unsure about where to seek care (see Table 5.10).

Interaction with Race. As a result of the bivariate analysis, a number of potential effect modifiers of the relationship between subject characteristics, race and delay attributed to each of the five reasons are evaluated. These include: a) for the concern with cost outcome - usual source of care, rural residence and self-perceived health status; b) for the distance or transportation outcome - education and assistance with transportation.

However, in the multivariate analysis, only one interaction remained. Rural residence modifies the relationship between race and delay in seeking medical care attributed to cost concerns. There are virtually no differences between the odds of white rural and non-rural elders in relation to delaying medical care because of concern with cost; using non-rural white elders as the reference category the odds for rural white elders in .97 (see Table 5.10). However, non-rural black elders have an odds ratio of only .34 that of white non-rural elders, while black elders who live in a rural county have an odds .68 that of white non-rural elders. Both groups of black elders are less likely than white elders to say that they postpone going to the doctor because of concern with the cost of a visit, and this is particularly true of elderly blacks living in a non-rural county.

Delay in Seeking Medical Care Attributed to Attitudinal Barriers

Table 5.11 displays the adjusted odds ratios and 95 percent confidence intervals for predisposing, enabling and need-for-care characteristics in relation to regularly delaying medical care because of attitudinal barriers. Two models were estimated: 1) delay attributed to the belief that going to the doctor would not do any good, and 2) delay attributed to the belief that problems would get better without intervention.

Predisposing Characteristics. The findings of the multivariate model are consistent with the findings of the bivariate analysis: elderly blacks are less likely than elderly whites to delay medical care because of attitudinal barriers. The odds that elderly blacks delay seeking medical care because of doubts about the efficacy of care is .47 that of elderly whites, and the odds that they will delay because of the belief that a problem will resolve without a visit is .51 that of elderly whites.

Other findings among the predisposing characteristics, in relation to delay attributed to the belief that problems would get better without a visit, include: being married which is associated with an increase in the odds (OR 1.44), on the other hand, being male (.78, 95% CI .58, 1.04) and increased education (OR for 12 years .57 that of 6 years of education) decrease the odds of delaying for this reason.

Enabling Characteristics. Income, which was highly associated with delay because of perceptions of barriers to access, does not alter the odds of delaying medical care because of attitudinal barriers. Insurance, also does not influence the decision to delay medical care for these reasons. However, usual source of care does. Lacking a usual source of medical

Table 5.11: Multivariate Analysis: Predisposing, Enabling and Need for Care Characteristics in Relation to Regularly Delaying Medical Care Because of Attitudinal Barriers.

Characteristic (n=3,746)	Going to the Doctor Will Not Do Any Good OR (95% CI)	Problem Will Get Better by Itself OR (95% CI)
Predisposing		
Age		
Race (Black=1)	0.47 (0.30, 0.71)	0.51 (0.37, 0.69)
Gender (Male=1)		0.78 (0.58, 1.04)
Martial Status (Married=1)	1.44 (1.01, 2.05)	
Living Alone		
Education		0.57 (0.41, 0.86)
Enabling		
Income		
$5,000[a]		
$5–9,999		
$10–19,999		
$20,000 +		
Insurance		
Medicare only		
Medigap		
Medicaid		
HMO		
Usual Source of Care		
Private[a]		
Other (OPD, Clinic)	1.37 (0.82, 2.30)	1.61 (1.10, 2.36)
None	3.25 (1.75, 6.07)	1.90 (1.13, 3.20)
Social Support		
No relative to turn to	1.87 (1.17, 2.98)	1.54 (1.08, 2.20)
No friend to turn to	0.60 (0.33, 1.09)	
No assistance when sick		
No assistance with transportation		1.80 (1.16, 2.40)
Rural Residence		
Need–for–Care		
Self Perceived Health		
Excellent./good[a]		
Fair	2.17 (1.45, 3.24)	1.81 (1.34, 2.45)
Poor	3.62 (2.29, 5.73)	2.33 (1.62, 3.34)
Illness Index		
Good health[a]		
Fair health		0.83 (0.61, 1.12)
Poor health		0.61 (0.45, 0.84)
Any disability (Yes=1)		

a – reference category

care is associated with more than a three-fold increase in the odds of delaying care seeking because of doubts about the efficacy of care (OR for believing a visit would not do any good is 3.25), and a nearly two-fold increase in the odds of delayed care seeking because of the belief that problems would resolve without intervention (OR for delaying because of the belief that problems would get better by themselves is 1.90). In the bivariate analysis, there was a weak association between identifying a clinic as a usual source of care and delaying medical care because of attitudinal reasons (see Table 5.6). In the multivariate analysis, elders who identify a clinic as a usual source of care have a small, but non-significant, increase in their odds of doubting the efficacy of care (OR 1.37, 95% CI .82, 2.30) and a stronger, and significant, increase in their odds of believing medical problems will get better without intervention (OR 1.61, 95% CI 1.10, 2.36).

Social support measures play a larger role in the two models of attitudinal barriers than in the three models of perceived access barriers. Elders without a supportive relative are more likely to delay for both attitudinal reasons (OR 1.87 and 1.54), while elders who *did not* receive assistance with transportation were 1.80 times more likely to attribute the cause of delay to the belief that a problem would get better by itself, as compared with those who did receive help with transportation.

Need for Care Characteristics. Once again, fair and poor self-ratings of health are strongly associated with delay. Elders in these categories increase their odds of attributing delay to attitudinal barriers (Table 5.11) as well as to access barriers (Table 5.10). For example, perceiving one's health as poor is associated with a 3.62 fold increase in the odds of delaying because of the belief that a visit would not do any good, as compared with perceiving one's health as excellent or good. Whereas, once again, the Illness Index has an opposite effect on delay; the poor health as measured by the Illness Index is associated with a decrease in the odds of delay (OR .61 comparing poor health with good health) because the problem would get better by itself. Self-perceived health and the Illness Index measure different attributes of the concept of health and affect the decision to seek care in different ways. Contrary to the bivariate analysis, in the multivariate model the presence of disability did not emerge as a significant influence on the odds of delaying because of attitudinal barriers.

ANALYSIS OF THE USE OF PHYSICIAN VISITS

Study Question: Does the pattern of physician visits differ for elders who delay medical care because of access concerns versus elders who delay medical care because of attitudinal reasons?

Figure 5.2: Direct Effects of Subject Characteristics and Delay on Physician Visits

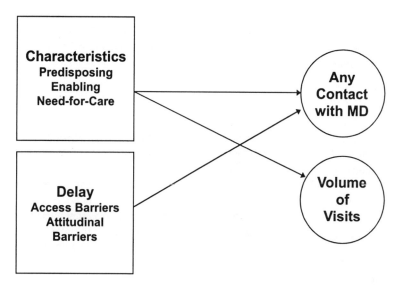

This section presents findings from the analysis of delay, predisposing, enabling and need-for-care characteristics on physician visits (see Figure 5.2). Estimations were made of the relationship between these variables and two outcomes measuring physician visits: *no* annual contact with a physician, and number of visits among *users* of care (those with one or more visits). The 'no contact' outcome is a dichotomous dependent variable and was estimated using logistic regression analysis, while the 'number of visits' is a continuous outcome and was estimated using ordinary least squares estimations; each outcome is presented separately in the bivariate and multivariate sections. As with the analysis of delay, the presentation of findings is as follows: (1) bivariate analysis, (2) adjustments for race, and (3) multivariate modeling.

Bivariate Analysis

The results of bivariate analysis are displayed on Table 5.12. Weighted, unadjusted odds ratios (OR) and 95 percent confidence intervals (95% CI) are shown for the five delay variables, as well as predisposing, enabling and need-for-care characteristics, in relation to the likelihood of having no physician contact during the year preceding the interview. Unadjusted beta coefficients and standard errors are reported for subject characteristics and delay variables in relation to the number of physician visits among users of care. For ease of interpretation, ORs whose 95% CIs do not contain unity and beta coefficients with a $p<.05$, are displayed in bold type.

Bivariate Analysis - No Annual Contact With a Physician

Delaying Medical Care. Five measures of delay are included in this analysis. There are three measures of delay attributed to perceived access barriers: (1) concern with cost, (2) unsure where to go for care, and (3) distance or transportation difficulties; and two measures of delay attributed to attitudinal barriers: (1) delaying because going would not do any good, and (2) delaying because the problem would get better by itself. As shown in Table 5.12, there is a weak association between perceptions of access and foregoing contact with a physician, however, the confidence intervals for these estimations contain unity. For example, delaying medical care because of concern with cost is associated with a 28 percent increase in the odds of foregoing contact with a physician (OR 1.28) however, the 95 percent confidence interval ranges from .94 to 1.74. On the other hand, delaying medical care because of attitudinal barriers is associated with a significant increase in the odds of *not* seeing a physician during the 12 months preceding the interview. Believing that a visit would not do any good increases the odds of no physician contact by two-fold (OR 2.04), while elders who delay because they believe a problem would resolve by itself have an odds of 1.62, compared with those who do not delay for this reason.

Predisposing Characteristics. Among predisposing variables, age and education have a statistically significant, but not substantive, association with physician contact; the odds of foregoing a visit for a 75 year old is .91 that of a 65 year old while the odds of 12 years of education are .95 that of 6 years of education. Being male is associated with a 27 percent increase in the odds of having no physician contact (OR 1.27, 95% CI 1.01, 1.58). Overall, none of the predisposing characteristics, including race, are strongly associated with this outcome.

Table 5.12: Weighted Bivariate Analysis of Physician Visits, Both Contact and Volume.*

Characteristic	NO Contact With Medical Care During Preceding 12 Months (n=3,746) Odds Ratio (95% Confidence Interval)	Number of Visits Among USERS of Care (n=3,016) beta coefficient (standard error)
Delaying Medical Care		
perceived barriers to access:		
Concern with cost	1.28 (0.94, 1.74)	0.05 (0.29)
Unsure where to go	1.37 (0.75, 2.51)	0.36 (0.54)
Distance or transportation	1.23 (0.75, 2.02)	**1.48 (0.56)[d]**
attitudinal barriers		
Going won't do any good	**2.04 (1.43, 2.92)**	0.26 (0.41)
Problem will get better	**1.62 (1.20, 2.19)**	−0.15 (0.31)
Predisposing Characteristics:		
Age[a]	0.91 (0.89, 0.92)	0.22 (0.12)
Gender (Male=1)	**1.27 (1.01, 1.58)**	−0.26 (0.15)
Race (Black=1)	0.90 (0.73, 1.11)	0.18 (0.16)
Married (yes=1)	0.96 (0.79, 1.17)	**−0.29 (0.15)[e]**
Living alone (yes=1)	1.13 (0.94, 1.36)	0.19 (0.14)
Education[b]	**0.95 (0.92, 0.97)**	**−0.06 (0.02)[d]**
Enabling Characteristics:		
Income		
$5,000[c]		
$5– 9,999	1.23 (1.00, 1.54)	−0.30 (0.18)
$10–19,000	1.07 (0.84, 1.37)	**−0.71 (0.22)[d]**
$20,000 +	1.03 (0.72, 1.47)	**−0.89 (0.22)[d]**
Insurance		
Medigap	0.88 (0.72, 1.06)	**−0.33 (0.15)[e]**
Medicaid	0.64 (0.39, 1.06)	**1.32 (0.34)[d]**
HMO	1.45 (0.92, 2.29)	**−0.52 (0.24)[d]**

Table 5.12 continued

Characteristic	NO Contact With Medical Care During Preceding 12 Months (n=3,746) Odds Ratio (95% Confidence Interval)	Number of Visits Among USERS of Care (n=3,016) beta coefficient (standard error)
Usual Source of Care		
Private[c]		
Clinic	**0.66 (0.50, 0.87)**	−0.11 (0.21)
None	**9.02 (6.54, 12.43)**	**−1.81 (0.48)[d]**
Social Support		
No relative to turn to	0.97 (0.76, 1.23)	0.44 (0.25)
No friend to turn to	0.94 (0.71, 1.24)	0.44 (0.25)
No assistance when sick	**2.60 (2.06, 3.28)**	**−1.30 (0.19)[d]**
No assistance with transportation	**1.38 (1.16, 1.65)**	**−1.11 (0.16)[d]**
Rural Residence	0.82 (0.65, 1.05)	**0.80 (0.17)[d]**
Need for Care Characteristics:		
Self Perceived Health		
Excellent/good[c]		
Fair	**0.61 (0.49, 0.75)**	**1.42 (0.17)[d]**
Poor	**0.23 (0.16, 0.34)**	**2.95 (0.27)[d]**
Illness Index		
Good[c]		
Fair	0.82 (0.66, 1.02)	**0.74 (0.19)[d]**
Poor	**0.44 (0.35, 0.55)**	**1.84 (0.18)[d]**
Disability (Any=1)	**0.34 (0.24, 0.47)**	**2.10 (0.21)[d]**

* OR whose 95% CI does not contain unity is displayed in bold type.
a – odds ratio compares a 75 year old with a 65 year old.   b – compares 6 years of education with 12 years
c – reference category   d – statistically significant at p<.01
e – statistically significant at p<.05

Enabling Characteristics. Income, insurance, usual source of care, social support and rural residence are included as enabling characteristics. Surprisingly, in this unadjusted analysis, income and insurance have no statistically significant association with physician contact. They do, however, influence volume of services used.

A lower proportion of elders who identified a clinic as a usual source of care forego all physician contact for a 12 month period, as compared with those who receive their care at private physician offices (OR .66). However, lacking a usual source of care is associated with a *nine* fold increase in the odds of having no physician contact as compared with elders who name a private physician office as their source of care (OR 9.02, 95% CI 6.54, 12.43).

The relationship between social support and no physician contact varies. Lacking supportive relatives and/or friends is not associated with physician contact. However, elders who did not receive instrumental support (no assistance when sick and no assistance with transportation) were more likely to forego annual physician contact (OR 2.60 and 1.38, respectively). Note that the bivariate analysis is not adjusted for health status.

Need-for-Care. All three measures of health status (self-rated health, Illness Index and presence of disability) are strongly associated with physician contact; as health status worsens the odds of foregoing any physician contact decreases. For example, poor self-rated health is associated with an odds ratio .23 that of excellent or good ratings (see Table 5.12).

Bivariate Analysis - Number of Physicians Visits Among Users of Care

The results of bivariate analysis for this continuous outcome are displayed on the right column in Table 5.12. These are beta coefficient estimates from a one factor regression analysis. Estimates that are statistically significant at the .05 level or below are highlighted in bold lettering.

Delaying Medical Care. Among the five measures of delay, only delay attributed to distance or transportation has a significant association with volume of physician visits. Interestingly, elders who attribute delay to transportation difficulties average an additional 1.48 visits per year. Branch and Nemeth (1985) also found that transportation difficulties were associated with an increase in the number of physician visits, suggesting that the more often the older individual goes to the doctor the more frequently he/she encounters problems with transportation.

Predisposing Characteristics. Among these characteristics, marital status and education are associated with a decrease in average number of physician visits; married elders average .29 fewer visits per year, while each year of education decreases the number of physician visits by .059. Age, gender, race and living alone did not have a statistically significant association with volume of physician visits.

Enabling Characteristics. Income is inversely related to number of physician visits; as income increases the average number of physician visits decrease. The availability of Medigap insurance decreases average number of annual visits by .325, while Medicaid insurance increases the number of annual visits by 1.32. Membership in a health maintenance organization is associated with one half fewer visits per year (-.523).

Among users of care, no usual source of care is associated with 1.8 fewer physician visits per year, while the average number of physician visits for elders who are seen at a clinic is virtually the same as for those seen at a private physician office. Older adults who did not receive assistance with illness or transportation averaged 1.3 and 1.1 fewer annual visits, respectively. Finally, rural residence is associated with an increase in the number of physician visits of nearly .8.

Need-for-Care. All three measures of health status are associated with an increase in the average number of physician visits. For example, elders who rate their health as poor average nearly 3 visits more than elders who rate their health as excellent or good.

Research Question: Does race mediate the use of physician visits?

Unadjusted and Adjusted Odds Ratios and Beta Coefficients for Race in Relation to Physician Utilization

To address this research question, the bivariate analysis was repeated adjusting for race. The results are displayed in Table 5.13. The unadjusted odds ratios and beta coefficients do not point to a significant association between race and physician visits (OR for contact is .90 and beta estimate for number of visits is .183). Looking at the 'no contact' outcome (first column of numbers on Table 5.13), it is evident that none of the delay variables, or the predisposing, enabling and need-for-care characteristics, confound the relationship between race and this outcome. Three variables potentially modify the relationship between race and foregoing physician visits and were explored further in the multivariate modeling. These include delay attributed to the belief that a visit would not do any good, gender, and self-perceived health status.

Table 5.13: Race and Physician Visits: Unadjusted and adjusted estimate of effect for race in relation to contact with a physician and volume of visits among users of care.*

	NO Annual Contact With Medical Care (N=3,746) OR (95% CI)	Number of Visits Among USERS of Care (N=3,016) beta (S.E.)
Estimate for Race, Unadjusted	0.90 (0.73, 1.11)	0.183 (0.157)
Estimate for Race, Adjusted for:		
Delaying Medical Care Because of:		
perceived barriers to access		
Concern with cost	0.90 (0.73, 1.11)	0.183 (0.157)
Unsure where to go	0.90 (0.73, 1.11)	0.185 (0.157)
Distance or transportation	0.90 (0.72, 1.11)	0.160 (0.156)
attitudinal barriers		
Going won't do any good	**	0.191 (0.157)
Problem will get better	0.91 (0.74, 1.12)	0.180 (0.157)
Predisposing Characteristics:		
Age	0.90 (0.73, 1.11)	0.181 (0.156)
Gender (Male=1)	**	**
Married (yes=1)	0.90 (0.73, 1.10)	0.154 (0.153)
Living alone (yes=1)	0.90 (0.73, 1.10)	0.191 (0.158)
Education	0.86 (0.70, 1.07)	**
Enabling Characteristics:		
Income	0.89 (0.72, 1.10)	**–0.093 (0.158)**
Insurance		
Medigap	0.84 (0.66, 1.05)	**0.066 (0.170)**
Medicaid	0.92 (0.74, 1.14)	**0.096 (0.156)**
HMO	0.91 (0.74, 1.12)	0.175 (0.261)
Usual Source of Care	0.89 (0.70, 1.13)	0.232 (0.168)
Social Support		
No relative to turn to	0.90 (0.73, 1.11)	0.189 (0.156)
No friend to turn to	0.90 (0.73, 1.12)	0.183 (0.157)
No help when sick	0.93 (0.75, 1.15)	0.144 (0.158)
No help with transportation	0.92 (0.74, 1.13)	0.120 (0.157)
Rural Residence	0.92 (0.74, 1.13)	0.113 (0.153)
Need–for–Care Characteristics:		
Self Perceived Health	**	**0.020 (0.148)**
Illness Index	0.91 (0.74, 1.13)	0.132 (0.154)
Any Disability (yes=1)	0.91 (0.74, 1.12)	0.159 (0.154)

* – bold numbers indicate variables that confound the relationship between race and the outcome.

** – interaction is statistically significant (at the $p<.05$ or below) therefore, adjusted OR is irrelevant.

The results displayed in the 'average number of physician visits' column show that income, insurance and self-rated health are weak confounders of the relationship between race and volume of services, however, the variances of the point estimates are too large for the relationship to be statistically significant. Gender and education modify the relationship between race and physician visits and were included, along with their interaction terms, in the multivariate modeling.

Summary of the Bivariate Analysis

Table 5.14 displays a summary of the bivariate analysis of physician utilization. Once again, plus signs indicate a positive association with the outcome while a minus sign indicates a negative association. Blank spaces indicate that an association was explored but no statistical or substantive significance was found; stars represent an interaction between the variable and race. Overall, in the bivariate analysis, there are only three significant relationships between delay and utilization. Delay because of distance or transportation increases average number of physician visits; delay attributed to the belief that the problem will get better by itself increases the odds of not seeing a physician for at least one year and, the effect of delay because of the belief that going would not do any good varies by race. Lacking a usual source of care increases the odds of not having any physician visits and decreases average number of physician visits among those with one or more visits; this pattern is the same for elders who did not receive any assistance from others for illness. The need-for-care measures decrease the likelihood that an older person would not have any physician visits and is associated with an increase the number of visits among users of care. There are a number of interactions which are evaluated in the multivariate analysis (see Table 5.14).

Table 5.14: Summary of Bivariate Analysis: Increase (+) or Decrease (–) in the Odds of Contact With a Physician and Volume of Visits Among Users of Care.*

Variables	NO Contact With Medical Care During Preceding 12 Months (n=3,746)	Average Number of Visits Among USERS of Care (n=3,016)
Delaying Medical Care		
perceived barriers to access:		
Concern with cost		
Unsure where to go		
Distance or transportation		
attitudinal barriers:		+
Going won't do any good	**	
Problem will get better	–	
Predisposing Characteristics:		
Age		
Gender (Male=1)	**	**
Race (Black=1)	**	**
Married (yes=1)		–
Living alone (yes=1)		
Education		**
Enabling Characteristics:		
Income		–
Insurance		
Medigap		–
Medicaid		+
HMO		
Usual Source of Care		
Clinic	–	
None	+	–
Social Support		
No relative to turn to		
No friend to turn to		
No assistance when sick		–
No assistance with transportation	+	–
Rural Residence		+
Need for Care Characteristics:		
Self Perceived Health	**	+
Illness Index	–	+
Disability (Any=1)	–	+

* – Note: bivariable results which revealed no change in the odds are left blank.

** – Interaction between race and variable in relation to the outcome.

Multivariate Modeling

Modeling of physician utilization began with all variables included and continued with efforts to pare down the models, beginning with variables that were not associated with the likelihood of any visit or with the volume of visits. Because the relationship between the delay variables and utilization is of great interest to this analysis, all five delay variables are included in the final model. Significant interactions from the bivariate analysis are examined as well. The final multivariate models are displayed on Table 5.15.

The findings for the multivariate logistic regression analysis of the likelihood of having no contact with a physician are discussed below, followed by the findings from the ordinary least squares estimation of average number of physician visits among users of care. As with all multivariate modeling, final estimations were conducted using SUDAAN software.

No Annual Contact With a Physician

Odds ratios and 95 percent confidence intervals for the variables included in the final model of physician contact are displayed in Table 5.15. A blank space indicates that the association between a given variable and the outcome was assessed, found not to have a significant association with the outcome, did not confound or modify the relationship between any other variable and the outcome and, consequently, was dropped from the final model.

Delaying Medical Care. Perceived barriers to access are not associated with the likelihood of foregoing physician contact during the course of a year. These findings suggest that perceptions of access *do not* influence entry into the health care system. This, however, is not the case for attitudinal barriers. The odds for elders who doubt the efficacy of a physician visit (regularly delay medical care because of the belief that going to the doctor would not do any good) in relation to *no* annual contact with a physician are more than doubled (OR 2.28). Doubts regarding the efficacy of medical care do seem to present a barrier to entry into the health care system.

Table 5.15: Multivariate Analysis: Delay behaviors, predisposing, enabling and need–for–care characteristics in relation to contact with physician (n=3,746) and volume of visits (n=3,016).

VARIABLE	NO Annual Contact with a Physician OR (95% CI)	Number of Visits Among USERS of Care beta (s.e.)
Delaying Medical Care Often:		
Because of Perceived Access Barriers:		
Concern with Cost	1.01 (0.62, 1.65)	–0.92 (0.38)[a]
Unsure where to go	0.77 (0.38, 1.56)	0.17 (0.57)
Distance or Transportation	1.00 (0.55, 1.78)	**1.30 (0.51)[a]**
Because of Attitudinal Barriers:		
Going won't do any good	**2.28 (1.48, 3.50)**	0.25 (0.46)
Problem will get better	1.45 (0.88, 2.40)	–0.40 (0.38)
Predisposing Variables		
Age		
Race (Black=1)	0.81 (0.63, 1.04)	0.23 (0.21)
Gender (Male=1)		–0.08 (0.20)
Interaction: Male*Black		**– 0.58 (0.27)[a]**
Marital Status (Married=1)		
Living Alone		
Education		
Enabling Variables		
Income		
$5,000[d]		
$5–9,999	1.11 (0.85, 1.44)	0.26 (0.20)
$10– 19,999	0.82 (0.60, 1.13)	0.26 (0.20)
$20,000+	0.70 (0.46, 1.07)	**0.46 (0.22)[a]**
Insurance		
Supplementary to Medicare	**0.76 (0.58, 0.98)**	
Medicaid		**0.73 (0.30)[b]**
HMO		
Usual Source of Care		
Private Physician[d]	**0.68 (0.50, 0.93)**	–0.16 (0.18)
Clinic	**6.93 (4.85, 9.91)**	–1.20 (0.36)[c]
None		
Social Support		
No relative to turn to		**0.44 (0.24)**
No friend to turn to		
No assistance when sick	**2.03 (1.61, 2.57)**	**–0.57 (0.18)[b]**
No assistance with transportation		**–0.56 (0.16)[b]**
Rural Residence		**0.66 (0.17)[c]**

Table 5.15 continued

VARIABLE	*NO* Annual Contact with a Physician OR (95% CI)	Number of Visits Among USERS of Care (beta, s.e.)
Need for Care Variables		
Self Rated Health Status[d]		
Excellent/Good		
Fair	**0.68 (0.54, 0.85)**	**1.00 (0.163)[c]**
Poor	**0.29 (0.19, 0.45)**	**2.17 (0.256)[c]**
Illness Index		
Good Health[d]		
Fair Health	0.98 (0.76, 1.26)	**0.45 (0.189)[a]**
Poor Health	**0.63(0.49, 0.81)**	**1.156 (0.178)[c]**
Disability (Any=1)	**0.79 (0.68, 0.92)**	**1.249 (0.219)[c]**
Intercept		3.245
R–square		0.154

* – bold numbers indicate statistically significant results.
a – p– value <.05
b – p–value <.01
c – p–value <.0001
d – reference category

Predisposing Characteristics. Variables that modified the relationship between race and contact with a physician in the unadjusted bivariate analysis (gender, attitudinal barrier, and self-perceived health) were not found to be statistically significant interactions in the multivariate analysis. Race has a weak, negative association with physician contact; the odds for elderly blacks foregoing annual contact with a physician is .81 that of elderly whites (95% CI .63, 1.04).

Enabling Characteristics. As income increases there is a trend for the odds ratio, in relation to no physician contact, to decrease. In other word, the higher the income the lower the odds of no annual physician contact. While the trend is in this direction, note, however, that the 95 percent confidence interval for the income estimates contain unity. Contrary to findings in the bivariate analysis, elders who have a Medigap type health insurance policy (supplementary to Medicare) are less likely to forego annual contact with a physician (OR .76) as compared with elders who do not have this type of private insurance. The availability of Medicaid insurance and enrollment in a Health Maintenance Organization were not found to have an effect on the odds of physician contact.

Compared with elders who receive their care at a private physician's office, those who receive their care at a clinic are less likely to forego an annual physician visit (OR .68). On the other hand, elders who lack a usual source of care have a nearly seven-fold increase in their odds of foregoing annual contact with a physician (OR 6.93).

Only one measure of social support was found to be associated with physician contact. Elders who received no assistance from another person for illness doubled their odds of having no annual contact with a physician, as compared with those who did receive assistance (OR 2.03). Lacking relatives, friends and assistance with transportation were not associated with an increase or a decrease in the odds of entry into the health care system.

Need-for-Care Characteristics. As with the bivariate analysis, all three measures of health status were found to have a significant effect on whether or not any physician visits were reported. As health status worsens (self-perceived and Illness Index) the odds of foregoing annual physician contact decrease (see Table 5.15). For example, the odds for elders who perceive their health as poor in relation to no physician contact is .29, as compared with those who perceive their health as excellent or good. This finding is consistent with the utilization literature which has established the importance of health status in predicting the utilization of medical care. Because of the strong relationship between self-perceived health status and delay, and the association between delay attributed to attitudinal barriers and physician contact, delay for these reasons was examined as a potential effect modifier of the relationship between self-rated health and physician contact, however, none was found. Attitudinal barriers neither confound nor modify the relationship between self-rated health and entry into the health care system.

Number of Physician Visits Among Users of Care

The right hand column on Table 5.15 displays the ordinary least squares (OLS) estimates of delay, predisposing, enabling and need-for-care variables on the number of physician visits among users of care. The model explains only 15.42 percent of the variance of volume of physician visits. Although in keeping with the findings of other researchers using the behavioral model, the amount of variance explained by this model does not improve upon previous findings (see for example, Wolinsky and Coe, 1984; Branch and Nemeth, 1985; Eve, 1988).

Delaying Medical Care - Interestingly, contrary to the bivariate findings, multivariate results reveal that delaying medical care because of concern with cost decreases average number of physician visits by nearly 1 visit (-.923); this finding is statistically significant at p05. On the other hand, consistent with the bivariate findings, elders who delay care-seeking because of distance or transportation average more than one additional visit per year (beta estimate is 1.30). This latter finding is in keeping with the work of Branch and Nemeth (1985) who found that older adults who experience transportation difficulties also use more medical care, perhaps because the more services one uses the greater the risk of exposure (difficulty getting to appointment). Although Branch and Nemeth (1985) found that concern with cost was given as a reason for failing to seek care, unlike these findings, no association was detected when the outcome variable was volume of physician visits.

Predisposing Characteristics - Age, marital status, household composition and education were not found to have a statistically significant association with volume of physician visits. However, a significant interaction was found between race and gender. Holding all other variables in the model constant, the average number of physician visits for black males, white males, black females and white females is as follows:

White females	=	3.24 visits per year
Black females	=	3.47 visits per year
White males	=	3.16 visits per year
Black males	=	2.81 visits per year

Adjusting for health status, elderly black males average the fewest number of physician visits per year while elderly black females average the most visits. Among white elders the average number of visits are nearly the same.

Enabling Characteristics - Enabling characteristics, which are often used as indicators of access, continue to play a role in determining number of physician visits in this elderly population insured by Medicare. Among the enabling variables, income, Medicaid insurance, and rural residence were found to be associated with an increase in the average number of physician visits. With regards to income, an annual income of 20,000 dollars or more seems to be a threshold; below that income level there are no significant differences as compared with an income of 5,000 dollars or less, however, elders who report an annual income that is 20,000 dollars or above, average nearly .5 additional visits. Those lacking a regular source of medical care report 1.2 fewer visits.

Findings having to do with the social support variables continue to hint of a complex relationship between type of social support and utilization of health care services. Those who lack supportive relatives average slightly more physician visits (.436) while elders who did not receive instrumental support (no assistance when sick or no assistance with transportation) experienced a decrease in average number of visits (.57 and .56 respectively). As mentioned in the discussion of the bivariate analysis, it is not clear whether elders who did not receive instrumental support needed or desired that support. However, this analysis adjusts for health status which presumably controls for need, but not desire, for assistance.

Need-for-care Characteristics. Not surprisingly, health status measures are highly significant in this analysis. The average number of physician visits increase as health status decreases. This is consistent for all measures of health and is also consistent with prior research examining utilization within the behavioral model framework. There were no statistically significant interactions between race and health status measures.

The multivariate analysis was repeated with only the need-for-care characteristics in the model (not shown). The results were quite interesting. As reported earlier, the full model explained 15.42 percent of the variance of volume of physician visits. The results of the reduced model (including only the need-for-care variables, i.e., self-rated health, Illness Index and disability) explained 12.66 percent of the variance of volume of physician visits; this means that the additional variables explained only an additional 2.76 percent of the variance. Despite the limited addition in explained variance, it remains important to include variables other than health status measures in a model of utilization. The beta estimates (or the estimate of effect) for these health status measures differed in the limited and full models. This is consistent with previous work by Evashwick and colleagues (1984) who also found that although predisposing and enabling variables were of minor predictive value compared with need variables, they confounded the relationship between need-for-care and utilization.

DIRECT AND INDIRECT EFFECTS

In this section, results from the multivariate analysis of delay and the multivariate analysis of physician utilization are combined in an effort to summarize the direct and indirect effects of subject characteristics (predisposing, enabling and need-for-care) on entry to the health care system (contact) and volume of services (number of visits among users). Typically, regression analysis examines only the direct effect of variables.

Bollen (1989) argues that consideration of each type of effect leads to a more complete understanding of the relationship between variables. The direct effect "is that influence of one variable on another that is not mediated by any other variable in a path model. The indirect effects of a variable are mediated by at least one intervening variable" (Bollen, 1989; p. 36). Ideally, it would be best to obtain estimates of direct and indirect effects using structural equations modeling. However, as discussed in Chapter IV, to do that presents the researcher with a choice of accounting for design effects and sample weights (e.g., by using SUDAAN software) or ignoring these effects and obtaining structural equations estimations with questionable variances. In view of this dilemma, a decision was made to analyze the data in two separate analyses, one with delay as the outcome variable, the second with physician visits as the outcome variable and delay included as explanatory variables, thus obtaining point estimates and variances that account for weights and design effects.

The following figures provide a schema of the characteristics that influence utilization of physician services, directly and/or indirectly via an intervening variable representing perceptions about access or efficacy. Each group of subject characteristic, intervening delay variable and outcome is shown in a separate figure, even so, the associations reflect estimates that were adjusted for all variables in the model (see Tables 5.10, 5.11 and 5.15).

Direct and Indirect Effects: Factors Associated with the Odds of No Physician Contact

The only delay variable found to have a statistically significant association with lack of annual physician contact was the belief that going to the doctor would not do any good (No Good). This is included as an intervening variable in the path diagrams represented in Figures 5.3 to 5.5.

Figure 5.3 (see below) illustrates the direct and indirect effects of predisposing, characteristics on the likelihood of having no contact with a physician during the year preceding the interview.

Figure 5.3: Direct and Indirect Effects of Predisposing Characteristics on No Contact with Physician

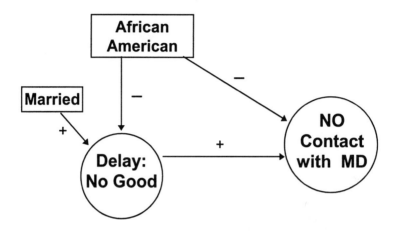

As illustrated in Figure 5.3, of the six predisposing variables examined (age, gender, education, marital status, household composition, and race), being married has an indirect effect on contact while race has both direct and indirect effects. Being married has a positive effect on the odds of delaying medical care because of the belief that a visit would not do any good, which in turn has a positive effect on the odds of foregoing any contact with a physician. On the other hand, elderly African-Americans are less likely to forego annual physician contact directly and indirectly via the negative effect of race (being black) on the belief that a visit would not do any good.

Figure 5.4: Direct and Indirect Effects of Enabling Characteristics
on No Annual Contact with Physician

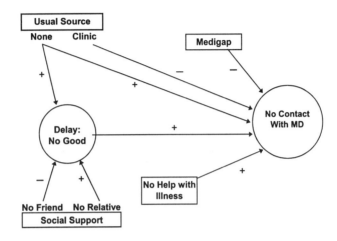

Among the enabling variables, characteristics that have a direct effect
include income, private insurance supplementary to Medicare (Medigap)
and no assistance for illness. Usual source of medical care influences
contact with a physician directly as well as indirectly through doubts about
the efficacy of care; two social support measures, lacking supportive
friends or relatives, have an opposite indirect effect on the odds of any
physician visits.

Figure 5.5: Direct and Indirect Effects of Need-for-Care
Characteristics on No Contact With Physician

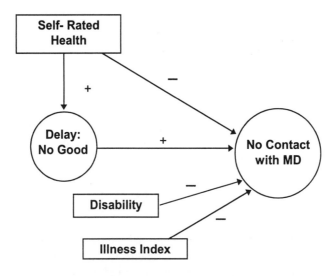

The presence of disability and chronic illness have a negative, direct
effect on the odds of not having any physician visits. On the other hand
self-rated health has a positive indirect effect and a negative direct effect
on this outcome. This seemingly paradoxical effect of self-rated health
needs to be better understood.

Direct and Indirect Effects: Factors Influencing the Volume of Physician Visits Among Users of Care

Two delay variables were found to have a statistically significant
association with the volume of physician visits among users of care. These
included concern with cost, and difficulty with transportation or distance
to physician. The associations are illustrated in the path diagrams presented in Figures 5.6 to 5.8. As with the earlier figures, the results
discussed reflect estimates adjusted for all variables in the model. As can
be seen in the figures below, factors that influence the volume of services
used by those already engaged in the system present a more complex
picture than determinants of entry.

Figure 5.6: Direct and Indirect Effects of Predisposing
Characteristics on Volume of Physician Visits

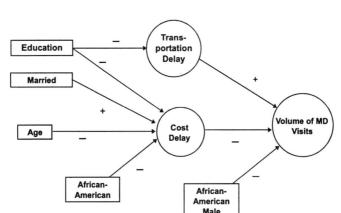

As shown in Figure 5.6, among the predisposing variables, age,
marital status and education have an indirect effect on the number of
physician visits via concern with cost (age and education have a negative
effect on concern with cost while marital status has a positive effect).
Education also influences number of visits through its negative effect on
delaying medical care because of transportation or distance difficulties. The
interaction between race and gender has a direct effect on volume of services.

Figure 5.7: Direct and Indirect Effects of Enabling Characteristics
on Volume of Physician Visits

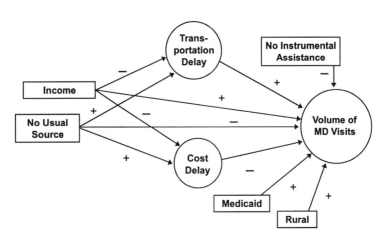

Having Medicaid insurance and lacking supportive relatives are associated with a positive, direct effect on the number of physician visits. The two measures of instrumental support (no assistance when ill and no assistance with transportation) have a *negative* and direct effect. Income and usual source of care have direct and indirect effects in a consistent and logical direction. Income affects volume of services indirectly via decreasing the odds of delaying medical care because of cost or transportation concerns as well as having a direct and positive effect. Elders lacking a usual source of care perceive more barriers to access and average fewer physician visits. Rural residence has a direct and indirect effect; living in a rural county is associated with a positive and direct effect on number of physician visits. In addition, living in a rural county modifies the relationship between race and delaying medical care because of concern with cost and has an indirect effect on this outcome.

Figure 5.8: Direct and Indirect Effects of Need-for-Care Characteristics on Volume of Physician Visits

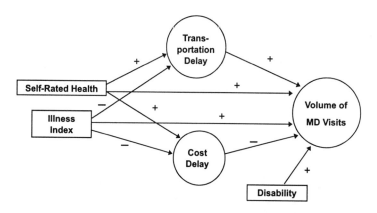

All three measures of health status have a strong direct effect on the number of physician visits. Self-rated health and Illness Index have opposite indirect effects on this outcome. Self-rated health has an indirect effect via its *positive* effect on delaying because of concern with cost and transportation. On the other hand, severity of illness, as measured by the Illness Index, has an indirect effect via its *negative* effect on these two intervening variables.

NOTES

1. Odds ratios were calculated as e^β where β is the logistic coefficient corresponding to the predictor variable being considered (in this case, not controlled for any other variables). The 95% confidence intervals were obtained using the formula $e^{(\beta \pm (1.96*SE))}$ where SE is the standard error associated with the logistic coefficient e^β. All SE for the unadjusted analysis were obtained using STATA software which accounts for proportional weighting and clustering.

2. While there are many ways to determine whether a given variable confounds the relationship of interest, in this bivariate analysis a conservative approach is taken whereby a variable is deemed to be a confounder if the odds ratio for the variable of interest (in this case it is race) changes by 10 percent or more.

VI

Conclusions

This chapter contains a discussion of the findings from this study. The first section provides a comparison of the hypothesized relationships versus those that emerged from the analysis. This is followed by a discussion of the limitations of the study in relation to the findings. Earlier studies and the conceptual model are then revisited and the relationship of the findings to the theoretical framework and prior research is examined. The generalizability of the findings and the implications for policy are then discussed followed by the conclusions.

HYPOTHESIZED VERSUS EMPIRICAL ASSOCIATIONS

Predisposing, Enabling and Need-for-Care Characteristics in Relation to Delaying Medical Care

Comparisons between the hypothesized and found directions of association between predisposing, enabling, and need-for-care characteristics in relation to delay in seeking medical care are displayed in Table 6.1. The plus signs indicate a positive association, minus signs indicate a negative association and question marks indicate conflicting previous findings or lack of sufficient prior research to provide guidance for hypothesized direction of effect. Under the findings column, lack of a positive or negative symbol indicates that no association was found.

Table 6.1: Comparisons of Hypothesized (H) Relationships Between Predisposing, Enabling and Need-for-Care Characteristics in Relation to Delaying Medical care and Findings (F).

Variable	Concern with Cost of Visit		Transportation or Distance Difficulties		Unsure of Where to Go		Problem Will Resolve by Itself		Going Won't Do Any Good	
	H	F	H	F	H	F	H	F	H	F
Predisposing										
Age	+	−			?		+		+	
Education	−	−	−		−		?	−	−	
Gender (Male=1)	−		−	−			?		+	
Household Composition (living alone=1)	+		+		+		−		−	+
Marital Status (married=1)	−	+	−		?		?	−	−	
Race(Black=1)	?	−	?		?		?		?	−
Enabling										
Income	−		−	−	−		?		?	
Health Insurance										
Medicare only[a]	−		−		−		?		?	
Medigap	−		+		−		?		?	
Medicaid	−		−		−		?		?	
HMO										
Source of Care										
Private[a]	−		+	+	?		?	+	?	
Public (Clinic)	+	+	+	+	+		+	+	+	+
None						+				+

Table 6.1 (continued)

Variable	Concern with Cost of Visit		Transportation or Distance Difficulties		Unsure of Where to Go		Problem Will Resolve by Itself		Going Won't Do Any Good	
	H	F	H	F	H	F	H	F	H	F
Social Support Network										
No Relative	–		–		–	–	?		?	
No Friend								–		+
Instrumental										–
No help when ill	–		–		–		?		?	
No help with transportation										
Residence (rural = 1)	?	***			?		?		?	
Need–for–Care										
Self-Rated Health	?				–		–		–	+
Health Index	?	–			–		–	–	–	
Physical Function	?			–	–		?		?	

a – reference category
*** – interaction with race

Expected and Unexpected Findings in the Association Between Predisposing Characteristics and Delay in Seeking Medical Care.
There are a number of differences between the associations hypothesized based on prior research and the findings from this study. Beginning with the predisposing variables, age was predicted to have a positive association with delay, however, once the analysis controlled for income, health status and social support, age was not associated with delay, with one exception: as age increased there was a decrease in the odds of delaying because of concern with cost. The work of Leventhal and Prohaska (1986) suggests that elders who attribute symptoms to aging are more likely to say they would cope by 1) waiting and watching, 2) accepting the symptoms, 3) denying or minimizing the threat, or 4) postponing or avoiding medical attention. Their research, along with that of Branch and Nemeth (1985), suggests that elders who attribute their symptoms to aging are more likely to forego a physician visit. The findings of this study support earlier research and suggest that perceptions of access and efficacy are not influenced by age per se, but rather by one's attitudes toward symptoms (symptoms generally being more prevalent as one ages), as well as by individual characteristics (e.g., education, health status or income). Additionally, Verbrugge (1985) found that taking actions to relieve symptoms was positively related to age and to education. This means that as age increases and education increases the likelihood of seeking medical visits in the presence of need (or symptoms) would increase. This finding is partially supported by the results of this study. While increased education was found to decrease the likelihood of perceiving barriers to access (concerns with cost and transportation difficulties), and increased age was found to decrease the likelihood of delay because of concern with cost, neither age nor education influences perceptions of efficacy.

It was expected that once characteristics such as income and social support were included in the analysis, marital status would not have an independent association with perceived barriers to access (married elders, in general, enjoy a higher income and have an accessible instrumental support person). On the whole, the findings were as expected. Surprisingly, however, married elders were more likely to delay because of concerns with cost. The reasons for this are not clear.

Although the direction of effect for race was not hypothesized, it was predicted that race would modify the relationship between the predictor variables and the outcomes. Overall, elderly African-Americans are less likely, than elderly whites, to say that they delay seeking medical care when they need to go. When the analysis holds factors such as income, education, and health status constant, black elders are less likely to report concerns with the cost of care, and less likely to question the efficacy of a physician visit. Although the reasons for the strong association between race and attitudinal barriers are not clear, white elders are more likely than black elders, to voice doubts regarding the efficacy of a visit as well as to voice the belief that health problems would resolve without intervention. This finding suggests that positive associations found previously between African-Americans and delay of medical care (for example, Weissman et al., 1991), may be attributed to issues such as socio-economic status and insurance, rather than race. The work of Garrett and colleagues (1993) suggests that African-Americans are more likely to desire state-of-the-art, intensive interventions at the end-of-life. This may reflect a strong belief in the efficacy of medical care, as well as a suspicion, resulting from many years of encountering racism, that decisions regarding how much care is given may be influenced by race rather than need.

As predicted, higher income is negatively related to delay because of cost and distance or transportation difficulties. This suggests that for elders with low income, financial barriers to access exist despite the availability of Medicare insurance coverage. This may be the result of a number of factors: not all physicians accept Medicare assignment, Medicare part B does not cover the entire cost of a physician visit, and out-of-pocket costs of medical care for elders have increased. In 1966, at the start of the Medicare program, out-of-pocket costs as a percent of elders' income was 15 percent. By 1977 it had decreased to 12.3 percent, however, during the next decade it increased, and by 1988 out-of-pocket costs for health care comprised 18.2 percent of the income of elderly people (Select Committee on Aging, U.S. House of Representatives, 1994). Thus, the out-of-pocket proportion of income was 20 percent higher at the time these data were collected than when Medicare was first implemented in 1966, and 50 percent higher than in 1977. The result of this inflation in out-of-pocket costs could contribute to elderly people's decision to delay medical care.

While higher socio-economic status decreases the odds of perceiving barriers to access, it has no effect on attitudinal reasons for delay. Income and education are not associated with delay attributed to doubts about the efficacy of a visit nor to the belief that problems would resolve without intervention.

Expected and Unexpected Findings in the Association Between Enabling Characteristics and Delay in Seeking Medical Care.
Contrary to the hypothesized effect, the availability of insurance in addition to Medicare (be it supplementary, Medicaid or a pre-paid plan) does not alter perceptions of access nor influences attitudes about the efficacy of care. This is particularly surprising for the concern with cost outcome since the expectation was that elders with supplementary insurance to Medicare or elders with Medicaid benefits would be less likely to have concerns about the cost of care. However, elders with Medigap insurance may be more likely to be seen at private physician offices which may, or may not, accept assignment. It is worth noting that while the availability of private supplementary insurance influences entry into the health care system and Medicaid coverage influences volume of services used (see Table 5.15), the availability of insurance in addition to Medicare does not alter *perceptions* of the health care system as being more or less accessible.

It was hypothesized that the availability of potential social support (network of friends or family) and realized social support (assistance with transportation or illness) would have a negative association with perceived barriers to access. With the exception of the finding that lack of a family network has a positive association with delay because of uncertainty about where to seek care, the remaining social support measures do not alter delay behaviors. It is interesting to note that while family network tempers discernment of where to seek care, the availability of a friend network does not seem to serve the same purpose. The literature suggests that the association between social support and attitudes toward medical care could go in either direction. These findings support that notion; effects do in fact go in both directions. Lacking a supportive relative *increases* the odds of delaying medical care because of doubts regarding the efficacy of a visit (delaying attributed to the belief that the problem will get better by itself and that going to the doctor would not do any good); on the other hand, lacking a supportive friend is associated with a *decrease* in delaying because of the belief that going would not do any good, but has no effect on the belief that a problem is self-limiting. This finding suggests that relatives and friends serve different functions in the process of seeking health care and that both measures must be examined separately, rather than combined, when investigating the relationship between social support and care seeking behaviors. Perhaps older adults who lack a supportive relative are unable to validate symptoms with another individual who would encourage them to seek medical care. Alternatively, Stoller (1993) found that people with larger support networks (it is not clear whether this network consists of friends, relatives or a combination) are less likely to interpret symptoms as serious medical problems. Stoller suggests several interpretations for this finding. First, social support may buffer the negative effects of symptoms, actually reducing their perceived intensity. Second, members of support networks may assist elders in meeting role obligations, thus reducing the visibility of incapacity. Finally, Stoller argues that network members may also serve as lay medical consultants, redefining the older person's initial assessments or suggesting treatment to alleviate symptoms.

It is unclear why receiving instrumental support (particularly assistance with transportation) does not lower the odds of delay because of distance or transportation difficulties. One would think that if transportation needs are being provided then the likelihood of encountering a problem with transportation would be lessened. However, an important limitation of this measure is that there is no accompanying assessment of need for transportation.

Elders who lack a usual source of care are more likely to perceive barriers to access and more likely to question the efficacy of a visit. Although the proportion of older adults who lack a usual source of medical care is relatively small (nearly 6 percent) it accounts for a large proportion of delayers. It is not clear from this research whether doubts regarding the efficacy of medical care and perceived barriers to access account for a lack of connection with a stable source of medical care, or the other way around. In an attempt to better understand who among this sample of older adults lacks a physician, an exploratory analysis was conducted that examined factors associated with no usual source of care. Descriptive statistics revealed that a larger proportion of black elders lack a usual source of medical care, as compared with white elders. However, in a multivariate analysis (which included education, supplementary insurance and income), the association between race and lack of a usual source of care disappeared. Although elders lacked a usual source of care tended to be black, poor, and living in Durham county they also had fewer years of education and lacked insurance supplementary to Medicare. Despite the inclusive insurance provided by Medicare to this population, elders who are disconnected with the health care system tend to be disproportionately of lower socio-economic status and African-American.

There is a positive association between a clinic as the site of the usual source of care and delay attributed to distance or transportation difficulties. This may speak to the location of clinics in relation to the residence of elders who are seen at the clinic. In order to explore whether rural residence influences the relationship between clinic as a source of care and delaying because of distance or transportation, a two-by-two table was constructed, stratified by rural residence, and odds ratios approximating the relative risk of delaying because of transportation difficulties were calculated for elders who received their health care at clinics. There were no differences in the odds for rural and urban elders suggesting that elders who live in a rural county, and who identified a clinic as a usual source of care, were no more likely to delay because of transportation difficulties than elders living in an urban county.

The average travel time for a physician visit is 19 percent longer for the elderly residing in non-metropolitan areas than for their metropolitan counterparts (Long and Settle, 1984). Yet "physicians' allowable charges under Medicare and, hence, the required coinsurance payments by the elderly are 20 percent lower in non-metropolitan areas for an identical service. Therefore, on average, waiting and travel time costs would represent a larger proportion of the full price confronting rural dwellers than they would for urban dwellers" (Long and Settle, 1984; p. 640). Consequently, it was hypothesized that rural elderly people would be more likely to delay for reasons of concern with cost and transportation difficulties as compared with urban elders. The findings revealed that while there was no independent effect of rural residence on delay, rural residence does modify the relationship between race and delay because of concern with the cost of care. There were no differences between the rates of delay because of cost for rural and urban elderly whites; however, while elderly blacks as a whole were less likely than elderly whites to delay for this reason, elderly blacks living in the urban county (Durham) had the lowest odds of delaying for this reason.

Expected and Unexpected Findings in the Association Between Need-for-Care Characteristics and Delay in Seeking Medical Care.
Another interesting difference between the expected and observed outcome is the relationship between health status and delay in seeking care. Three measures of health status were included in this study, with each measuring a different aspect of health: 1) self-rated health, 2) the presence of disability in performing activities of daily living, and 3) the Illness Index (which includes the presence and severity of five chronic illnesses). In the bivariable analysis, all three measures were associated with delay, however, when the three measures were included simultaneously in the multivariate analysis, the presence of disability was not associated with delay. On the other hand, self-rated health and the Illness Index had

opposite effects on delay in seeking medical care. It was hypothesized that fair and poor health would be associated with a decreased likelihood of delaying medical care. This was found to be only partially true. The worse the self-rating of health (in particular self ratings of poor health) the more likely elders were to perceive barriers to access as well as to question the efficacy of a visit. Self-rated health provides a subjective measure of the influence of illness and disability, and suggests a perceived need for care that the medical care system cannot adequately address. On the other hand, as the presence and severity of medically diagnosed illness increases (as measured by the Illness Index) the likelihood of delaying medical care, because of perceptions of access and because of perceptions of efficacy, decreases. This suggests that elders with serious medical illness do not delay physician visits in the presence of a perceived need for care. As noted in Chapter IV, a limitation of the Illness Index is that it does not include arthritis, a leading cause of chronic illness and disability among the elderly, it does, however, include medical illnesses such as diabetes, heart disease and cancer.

Rating one's health as poor has been associated with an increase in the likelihood of mortality among healthy (Schoenfeld et al., 1994), as well as impaired (Mossey and Shapiro, 1982), elderly community residents. Consequently, this finding is surprising and particularly worrisome. Even so, elders who rate their health as poor may very well have a rational basis for their remarks. They may reflect on the cost and the difficulty of getting to a physician, or, from prior experience, they may know that the physician cannot alleviate all their symptoms leaving them uncertain about where to go next to seek help. Conversely, elders who are in poor health as measured by the Illness Index have been given their diagnosis by a doctor consequently, they are better connected with the health care system and know where to go for care, and possibly how to get there; these people are not self-diagnosed.

Objective indicators, such as the Illness Index, can be considered to measure 'need' for health care, whereas subjective indicators can be said to measure 'demand' for health care (Wan, 1989). Therefore, it is not surprising that objective and subjective measures would predict perceptions of access differently. Thus, the presence of 'medicalized' illness promotes perceptions of efficacy and access with respect to the health care system, whereas a self-awareness of ill health (self-ratings of poor health), that may or may not be directly related to medically diagnosed illness, promotes a sense of frustration with barriers to access, as well as doubts concerning the capacity of medical intervention to alleviate problems.

Much of the illness experienced by elderly people involves chronic conditions. In particular, elders who suffer from debilitating, non-life threatening conditions such as arthritis, may have "an abundance of prescribed and non-prescribed medications and other treatment resources that must be gone through before they can declare themselves in need of additional social and medical resources (Alonzo, 1986; p. 1,307)." Furthermore, repeated reports of similar symptoms "not only fails to bring new information but can be seen as complaining or malingering (Schlesinger, 1993; p. 256)" by the physician. It is beyond the scope of this research to fully disaggregate the dynamics of why elders who perceive their health to be poor, and are high users of health care services, nonetheless report higher rates of delay behaviors. An examination of this process would be helped by analysis of longitudinal data from the Piedmont Health Survey of the Elderly.

Perceived Access or Attitudinal Barriers and Subject Characteristics in Relation to Physician Utilization.

Table 6.2 displays both the predicted and found directions of effects for the physician utilization outcomes.

Expected and Unexpected Findings in the Association Between Delay in Seeking Medical Care and Physician Visits. The most salient finding in this part of the analysis is that perceptions of access do not inhibit entry into the health care system while attitudinal barriers do; namely, those who attribute delay to concern with cost, distance or transportation difficulties or uncertainty about where to seek care, are no more likely than non-delayers to refrain from any contact with a physician. On the contrary, older adults who doubt the efficacy of a visit are more likely to avoid a visit altogether. However, perceptions of access do alter the volume of physician visits; elders who delay because they are concerned with the cost of care have fewer physician visits over the course of a year. These findings suggest that attitudes about health care services influence entry into the system, while perceptions of access influence volume of services. The findings support Donabedian's (1973) assertion that service use after initial entry is influenced by need, physician practice patterns and other socio-demographic variables. Medicare health insurance has helped to remove access barriers to initial entry, however, it has not fully removed barriers to volume of services. While it is beyond the scope of this research to determine definitively whether visits missed because of concern with cost were necessary or unnecessary visits, the finding of a statistically significant negative association between cost concerns and number of visits, while holding constant health status measures, suggests that visits missed were needed.

Table 6.2: Comparison Between Hypothesized (H) Relationships and Findings (F): Delay Medical Care, Subject Characteristics and Physician Visits.

VARIABLE	NO Physician Contact During the Preceding 12 Months		Number of Visits Among USERS of Care	
	H	F	H	F
Delay Attributed to:				
Access Barriers				
Concern with cost	?		–	–
Transportation or distance	?		–	
Unsure where to go for care			–	
Attitudinal Barriers				
Problem will resolve without intervention	+	+*	–	
Going to the doctor won't do any good	+	+	–	
Predisposing				
Age	–			
Education	–			
Gender (Male=1)	+		?	**
Household Composition (Living Alone=1)	?		+	
Marital Status (Married=1)	–		–	
Race (Black=1)	?	–	?	**
Enabling				
Income	–		?	+
Health Insurance	–			
Medigap		–	+	+
Medicaid			+	
HMO			?	
Source of Medical Care				
Private	–		+	
Public/Clinic	–	–	+	
None	+	+	–	–
Social Support Network				
No Relatives	–		?	+
No Friends	–		?	
Instrumental			+	
No help when sick	–	+		–
No help with transport	–			–
Residence (rural = 1)	?		?	
Need–for–Care				
Self–Rated Health	–	–	+	+
Physical Function	–	–	+	+
Illness Index	–	–	+	+

* – odds ratio contains unity

** – Interaction between race and volume of visits: black males had lowest number of visits, black females highest number.

The results include a puzzling association between delay attributed to transportation or distance difficulties and an increase in the number of physician visits. A possible explanation for this paradoxical finding is the direction of causality: elders who visit a physician more often have more opportunity for exposure (transportation difficulty). Although this finding is consistent with that of other investigators (for example, Branch and Nemeth, 1985), because these data are cross-sectional this study cannot clarify the underlying process for this finding. Longitudinal data are needed to understand the effect of transportation difficulties on utilization.

Expected and Unexpected Findings in the Association Between Predisposing, Enabling, and Need-for-Care Characteristics and Physician Visits. This study found that elderly African-Americans are more likely than elderly whites to have at least one physician visit during the course of a year; however, race interacts with gender to influence volume of services. Holding constant health status, as well as other indicators of physician utilization, being black and male is associated with fewer visits to a physician. Although white males average slightly fewer visits than white females, the differences are larger for black males and females. Studies that examine utilization of health care services by the elderly need to account for this interaction between race and gender.

Income and health insurance continue to play a role in entry to the system and volume of services used. Interestingly, while income does not influence the likelihood of contact with a physician, higher income is positively associated with number of physician visits. This suggests that among the elderly, financial factors do not pose a barrier to entry into the health care system, but rather, modify volume of use. The availability of insurance supplementary to Medicare (Medigap) increases the likelihood that an elder would have at least one physician visit during the course of a year, however, it does not influence extent of physician visits. Rice and McCall (1986) suggest that the causal association between volume of services and the availability of Medigap goes in both directions; in other words, elders who use more services are more likely to purchase a Medigap policy, consequently, holders of a Medigap policy are more likely to use more services. These findings do not support that assertion. While the availability of a Medigap policy increases the odds that some contact will be made with a physician, it does not seem to alter the number of visits once entry is gained. Medicaid, however, does not alter the odds of entry but does have a positive association with the number of visits once an elder is in the system.

Elders who lack a stable connection with the health care system are more likely to avoid any contact with a physician and average fewer physician visits during the course of a year. These are the elders who are at greatest risk for exacerbation of chronic illness as well as for loss of opportunity for early detection and preventive services, such as mammography and influenza vaccines.

Social support has little effect on entry into the system. Those lacking a network of supportive friends or relatives are no more likely to forego contact with a physician than those having one or more support persons. Whereas, lacking supportive relatives is associated with an increase in the number of physician visits. The results of the instrumental support measures were contrary to the hypothesized effects. Lacking assistance for illness is associated with an increase in the likelihood of having no annual contact with a physician, while lacking assistance with illness and with transportation are associated with a decrease in the volume of visits. So that, elders who do not receive instrumental support are less likely to have any physician visit, as well as fewer physician visits among those with one or more visits.

Living in a rural county is associated with an increase in the number of physician visits but does not alter the odds of a first visit. The reasons for this are not clear, however, there are a number of possible explanations. First, the area from which the sample was drawn does not offer a typical rural/urban dichotomy. Shortly after the 1986/87 interviews were completed, one of the counties included in the rural category had been designated as a metro county. In addition, the presence of major medical centers, as well as health clinics, in fairly close proximity make access less of an issue as would be the case for more isolated rural counties. These explanations point to a measurement problem with the rural variable, but do not explain the differences in utilization.

Health status is highly predictive of contact with, and volume of, medical services. These findings are as expected and support prior findings which concluded that, in this well insured population, measures of need rank as the first and foremost contributors to explained variance in utilization of services (Hulka and Wheat, 1985), as well as entry to the system.

LIMITATIONS OF THE STUDY

Data for this research are cross-sectional, consequently, it is beyond the scope of this study to establish causality. Delay behaviors as well as utilization patterns are recalled for the same time period. As a result, it is not possible to determine whether delay 'caused' the utilization pattern or whether recollections regarding utilization influenced recollections of delay. While statistical estimation techniques are available that would account for the correlation between delay and utilization, they do not allow for the estimation of simultaneous equations while at the same time accounting for design effects and sampling weights. A two-staged least squares estimation was attempted but results were illogical; the results from logistic regression were more conservative and are the ones reported in this study. Longitudinal data are needed to more fully elucidate the relationship between perceptions of access and attitudinal barriers and health services utilization.

Some health problems faced by elderly people are self-limiting and some problems do not respond well to medical intervention. In this study, it is not possible to determine when delaying for these reasons makes good use of self-care and is appropriate decision making, and when delaying for these reasons places the health of the older individual in jeopardy. An attempt is made to account for the appropriateness of the decision by defining delay only when it is reported to occur on a frequent basis and by simultaneously controlling for health status using several different measures of health.

The concept of appropriate health care utilization for elderly people, with neither overuse nor underuse, is a limitation of this study. Not all would agree that elderly people who are out of annual contact with a physician are under-utilizing the system, however, judging the appropriateness or consequences of omitted visits among users is beyond the scope of this study. Only the crude variable of reported utilization is available for this analysis. In an attempt to minimize this problem, the study differentiates between any contact with a physician and number of visits among users of care, while simultaneously controlling for health status.

Measurement of social support presents another limitation to the findings. The lack of information about attitudes held by friends and family members limits the ability to draw conclusions regarding the influence of a social support network on care seeking behaviors. Additionally, lack of information regarding the need for instrumental support, be it assistance for illness or transportation, also limits the ability to examine the role of instrumental support on the decision to seek medical care.

In this study, delay and need for physician visits are determined by individual perceptions. An individual who does not recognize a "need" for care would deny instances of delayed care seeking. This may explain why gender was not found to be a significant predictor of delay, or the lower rates of delay among African-American elders. Another significant limitation is the lack of direct observation of delay behaviors. Because this study was based on subject recall the meaning of occasional delay versus often delay may not be consistent for all participants of the study.

Another limitation has to do with measurement of one of the delay outcome variables. Specifically, the following questionnaire item: "were you unsure about where to go for help?" Using delay attributed to uncertainty about where to seek care as a dependent variable resulted in a less than satisfactory model. Uncertainty about where to seek care can arise from a number of factors, each of which may be related to a different set of explanatory variables. There are several possible explanations as to why elders may be unsure about where to seek medical care: 1) perhaps the individual has no connection with a physician and does not know to whom to go, 2) alternatively, elders who are so well connected that they regularly see many different physicians, may be confused about which physician to go to for a particular problem, or 3) elders who seen multiple physicians for chronic problems, that often lack easy resolutions, may really not know where to go next for help with their symptoms. Each explanation implies a different set of interventions. Investigators wanting to explore this issue need to consider further refinement of this measure.

RELATIONSHIP OF THE FINDINGS TO THOSE OF EARLIER STUDIES AND THE CONCEPTUAL MODEL

Racial differences in access to and utilization of health care services:

Escarce et al. (1993) found that, despite greater severity of illness, black elders were less likely to receive technologically advanced medical services; that race may exacerbate the impact of other barriers to access, and that racial differences in use of medical services persisted even when comparisons were made among elders of similar socio-economic backgrounds. This study found no racial differences in entry into the health care system, however, gender and race interact to modify volume of services; older black women average more physician visits than any other group while older black males average the fewest. Nonetheless, the types of services received, the intensity and level of technology, cannot be determined by this research. The likelihood of a medical encounter and the volume of encounters do not differ by race, however, more research is needed to determine whether the intensity and type of services differ by race, or by place of service. A third of elderly blacks receive health care services at a clinic, while more than three-fourths of elderly whites are seen at a private physician office. While these differences are not associated with differences in the odds of having any physician encounter or the number of visits, there may be, as the work of Escarce and colleagues (1993) suggests, differences in recommended treatments or procedures that may, or may not, be justified clinically.

This study found, as did Gibson and Jackson (1992), that black elders are more likely to live in families with limited economic resources. While income did not influence the odds of entry into the health care system, higher income was associated with more physician visits. Because a larger proportion of black elders live in poverty, the effects of income on will disproportionately affect this group of elders.

Two decades ago, Salber and colleagues (1976) concluded that, despite notable achievements by Medicare in providing access to hospital care for minority groups, the program had been less successful in other areas, namely physician services. Dr. Salber and colleagues found that elderly blacks had fewer physician visits despite being in poorer health. During that same period of time, Davis (1975) questioned the Medicare program's equal treatment and unequal benefits: "holding constant for health status, income, welfare status, education, availability of physicians, age and sex composition of the elderly population, low-income elderly blacks in the South have half as many physician visits as comparable whites." Davis did not find significant differences by race outside the South.

The findings of this research, using data from a population similar to Dr. Salber's sample, and gathered more than a decade later, demonstrates a marked change in the effect of Medicare on the ability of elderly southern blacks to access medical care. Not only do elderly black women average more physician visits per year, but elderly blacks are also less likely to report access barriers to services, and are less likely to avoid medical care because of doubts regarding the efficacy of care as compared with whites. However, the group with the fewest physician visits remains elderly black men. What has not changed since the early 1970's is the fact that more elderly blacks live in poverty, and more elderly blacks receive their care in clinics as opposed to private physicians' offices. Interestingly, the proportion of elders who do not have a usual source of care has remained constant. In both studies, approximately 7 percent of elderly blacks and 5 percent of elderly whites lacked a usual source of care.

Escarce and colleagues (1993) suggest that race modifies the relationship between access barriers and utilization of medical services, and Jackson and colleagues' (1982) "double jeopardy" hypothesis supports the assumption that factors such as economic status, health insurance coverage and perceived health status may interact with race in explaining utilization patterns. All these interactions were assessed and none was found to be statistically significant. Poverty, lack of insurance and poor self-ratings of health are more prevalent among elderly African-Americans, these factors do not, however, influence utilization differently for blacks than for whites. The reason for the interaction between gender and race is not clear. Perhaps elderly black women of this cohort experience poorer health (unmeasured by this research), or they have learned how to use the system more effectively.

Keith and Jones (1990) suggest that affordability is more of a problem for elderly blacks than whites, however, this was not found to be so for perceptions of affordability. Despite the lower income reported by elderly blacks, they are much less likely to attribute delay to concerns with cost. This finding persisted after usual source of medical care was held constant.

The findings of this research suggest that it is not race per se which accounts for differences in utilization, but rather factors that are more prevalent among black or white elders (for example, low income, illness or insurance status). However, there are differences in the way elderly African-Americans and elderly whites view the potential benefits (or lack of) resulting from an encounter with a physician. The reasons for these differences cannot be fully elucidated by this research.

Delaying Medical Care

There is a small, but significant, proportion of elderly people who avoid contact with the health care system because they question its efficacy. Stoller (1982) suggested that elders may ignore warning signs of serious conditions if they attribute them to aging. While increased age was not found to be associated with delay of medical care, attitudes regarding the efficacy of a visit were associated with delay and subsequent avoidance of any contact with a physician.

The present study found, as did Stoller (1982), that more than a third of elderly people reported putting off going to a doctor when they needed to go. Slightly more than 12 percent often delay going to a doctor, while another 27 percent occasionally put off care. Branch and Nemeth (1985) also found that 17 percent of elders in their study failed to visit a doctor when they perceived a need, and that attitudinal reasons accounted for 12 of the 17 percent. While previous studies did not examine delay among black elders, these findings suggest that while the prevalence of delay does not differ by race, reasons for delay do differ.

Utilization of medical care

High utilization of medical care among elderly people has been attributed primarily to health status and need for care (see Krause, 1990; Counte and Glandon, 1991; Kelman and Thomas, 1988; Wolinsky and Coe, 1984). This is confirmed by this study which found that health status indicators of need-for-care were responsible for more than 80 percent of the explained variance of volume of services used.

Approximately 19 percent of elders reported no annual contact with a physician. This is consistent with previous research (see for example, Branch and Nemeth, 1985; Shapiro and Roos, 1985; and National Center for Health Statistics, 1990). Factors associated with avoidance of any visit include lack of a stable connection with a physician and doubts regarding the efficacy of care.

This study supports the assertion that entry to the system and volume of services are two distinct concepts with different determinants (Donabedian, 1973; Penchansky and Thomas, 1981; Wolinsky, 1990). Among elders, perceptions of access do not inhibit entry but do influence volume of services used, while perceptions of efficacy do inhibit entry but do not influence extent of use. It would be interesting to see whether these hold for other segments of the population, for example children , who do not enjoy the benefits of nearly universal health care coverage.

This work contributes to the doubts voiced by other researchers regarding the utility of the Behavioral Model in explaining health care utilization by an older population (see for example, Krause, 1990). While this model provides a useful means of categorizing characteristics to be included in a model of utilization, it is clearly lacking some important factors which contribute to health-seeking behaviors as well as utilization itself. The use of longitudinal data, the inclusion of some measure of physician practice patterns, as well as prior utilization, may enhance the ability of this model to explain the extent of medical care use by the elderly.

This research advances theory by the inclusion of perceptions of access to and attitudes toward medical care as intervening variables between predisposing, enabling and need-for-care characteristics and utilization. The results of this study suggest the presence of factors that influence utilization indirectly via perceptions held by elders regarding the accessibility and efficacy of the system. It would be useful to discern the experiences that lead elders to question the efficacy of health care, particularly if these doubts result in avoidance of opportunities for preventive services, screening services or monitoring of chronic illness.

GENERALIZABILITY OF THE FINDINGS

Data from this study come from one region of the Southern United States, thereby limiting its generalizability. However, taken in context with findings from two similar studies (see for example, Stoller, 1989; Branch and Nemeth, 1985), the ability to generalize beyond the Piedmont region of North Carolina are strengthened somewhat. The prevalence of delay, as well as the prevalence of foregoing annual physician contact, are similar for this study and the two others cited. This is suggestive of a phenomenon that goes beyond a regional finding.

Unlike many previous studies, this investigation included a large component of African-American elders, and examined predictors of both contact with, and extent of use of, physician services. While these findings cannot be generalized to African-Americans living in other regions of the country, they do suggest differences in the way elderly blacks and elderly whites view medical care. The lack of additional elderly minority voices in this sample (for example, Native Americans, Asians or Hispanics) preclude the ability to generalize these findings to other elderly minority groups.

The proportion of subjects unavailable for health surveys increases with advancing age among those 65 and older (Fitti and Kovar, 1987; Herzog and Rogers, 1988), making it most difficult to obtain information directly from the oldest and frailest (Magaziner, 1992). Typically, a proxy respondent is obtained for subjects who are unable, or unwilling, to complete a survey. In the Piedmont Health Survey of the Elderly, proxy questionnaires were developed that did not include the sequence of questions measuring delay, consequently, it was necessary to drop proxy respondents from this study. This has implications for the generalizability of the findings from this study. The findings can be generalized to older adults who live in the community and who make their own decisions about seeking medical care. This precludes the ability to generalize the findings to elderly community residents who may not make their own decisions about seeking medical care (e.g., the very frail or confused).

IMPLICATIONS FOR POLICY

Rapid increases in expenditures for the Medicare program are motivating policy makers to search for ways to contain costs. For the elderly, a consequence of health care cost inflation is that health care costs are consuming an ever greater proportion of their income. If present trends continue, the elderly will soon pay out-of-pocket costs representing more than one fifth of their income. As out-of-pocket costs increase, so do concerns that the cost of a physician visit may result in a greater likelihood of putting off or neglecting to seek needed physician visits, a concern that affects, disproportionately, older adults living in poverty.

As policy makers debate various plans for health care reform, there are a number of lessons to be learned from older Americans who enjoy nearly universal health care coverage. First, it is important to consider that availability of insurance is a necessary, but not sufficient condition to seeking medical care; *perceptions* of access and the belief in the efficacy of care also affect use. If it is the intent of health policy to increase the use of preventive and early detection services such as screening mammography or influenza vaccines among older Americans, then service coverage as well as public education must go hand in hand. For example, influenza and associated illnesses are a leading cause of morbidity and mortality among the elderly population. In the spring of 1993 the influenza vaccine became a covered service under Medicare Part B. By itself, the incorporation of vaccines into entitlement programs may not significantly increase immunization rates. Attention must be paid to older adults who avoid contact with the health care system because they harbor doubts about the efficacy of care, or because they lack a stable connection with a health care provider. Financial access must accompany public awareness and education regarding the potential benefits associated with a health policy initiative, such as influenza immunizations for older Americans.

Second, Donabedian (1972) contends that the proof of access is use of services and that access can be measured by the level of use in relation to need. Further, he states that accessibility is more than availability of resources. "It comprises those characteristics of the resource that facilitate or obstruct use by potential clients" (p. 57). The achievements resulting from health care policy for elderly Americans have gone a long way to equalize access to Medical Care for all elders. As this study found, access barriers no longer prevent elderly persons from making an initial contact with a physician. However, efforts at paring down the Medicare budget, which would increase copayments or deductibles, could result in financial access re-emerging as a significant deterrent to use, disproportionately affecting the poor and the ill. As shown by these findings, *perceptions* of barriers to financial access alter care seeking behaviors and utilization.

Third, insurance in addition to baseline coverage increases the probability that at least one annual health care visit will be made, while higher income is associated with a greater extent of physician use. In addition, perceptions of financial barriers to medical care result in fewer annual physician visits. In other words, even among this well insured group of Americans, financial factors continue to moderate the use of medical care.

Finally, while racial disparities in treatment decisions for white and African-Americans have been noted, elderly blacks are no more likely than white elders to perceive financial or transportation barriers to seeking medical care. In fact, elderly African-Americans are less likely than elderly whites to doubt the efficacy of medical care or to believe that their health problems would resolve without medical interventions. This suggests that any disparity in the type and amount of medical interventions received by elderly African-Americans is not because black elders neglect to seek care for symptoms nor because they doubt the efficacy and importance of an intervention.

CONCLUSIONS

This work represents an effort to study the factors associated with the decision to delay or forego needed medical care, and the association of that decision with utilization of services. Given some of the limitations of the approach, both conceptually and methodologically, the findings are nevertheless useful insofar as they provide a better understanding of health care utilization by the elderly.

Three main questions of interest were addressed by the study. These include:

Who delays seeking medical care when there is a need to go, and why?

Does the pattern of physician visits differ for elders who delay medical care because of access concerns versus elders who delay medical care because of attitudinal reasons?

Does race mediate perceptions of access to or utilization of medical care?

The data reveal that older adults who lack a stable connection with the health care system (those who do not have a usual source of medical care), and older adults whose illness may be difficult to address by traditional medical interventions (those who rate their health as poor) are more likely to postpone or neglect to seek medical care. In addition, although Medicare health insurance for older Americans has helped to remove financial barriers to entry into the health care system it has not fully removed barriers to extent of physician use. Holding constant health status, as well as other indicators of utilization, older Americans living in poverty (annual income less than $5,000) average fewer physician visits as compared with those enjoying a higher income ($20,000 or more annually).

Reasons for delaying medical care included two categories: perceived barriers to access (including cost concerns, transportation or distance difficulties and uncertainty about where to seek care) and attitudinal barriers (including the belief that a problem is self-limiting and would resolve without intervention, and the belief that a visit would not be beneficial). The findings suggest that patterns of physician utilization differ for those who delay medical care because of access concerns versus elders who delay medical care because of attitudinal barriers. Doubts about the potential benefit of a physician visit influence entry into the health care system, while cost concerns decrease the number of physician visits among users of care.

Race does mediate the decision to delay medical care, but in an unexpected way. Race has no independent effect on the decision to delay medical care because of perceived financial or logistical access, however, race has an independent effect on delay because of attitudinal barriers; elderly whites are more likely than elderly blacks to neglect or postpone physician visits because of doubts about the potential efficacy of medical care.

In conclusion, the Medicare program has been tremendously successful in enabling elderly Americans to access medical care, however, income continues to be an important predictor of the volume of services used. In addition, *perceptions* of financial barriers also decrease the extent of utilization. Consequently, attempts to ease financial strains on the Medicare system by increasing the financial burdens of older adults will have a disproportionate effect on those of lower socio-economic status. Finally, while Medicare insurance is necessary for elders to access the health care system it is not sufficient. Attitudes and beliefs about the benefits of medical care also play a role in the decision to seek needed medical care among older adults.

APPENDIX

Appendix: Rationale behind hypothesized effects in Table 3.5 of Chapter 3.

Predisposing Characteristics

1) Studies examining the relationship between age and use of medical care have shown that this relationship is not linear (Wolinsky, 1990; Jackson and Gibson, 1992). The use of health care services by age follows an inverted 'J' distribution with use of services rising for the 'middle old' and decreasing for the 'oldest old'. On the other hand, while health status variables explain a significant amount of the variation in the use of health care services, they nevertheless provide only partial controls for the individual's state of health. Among the elderly, the prevalence of chronic illness tends to increase and general health status commonly worsens as people grow older. Accordingly, the age variable in the utilization equation may be viewed as an additional indicator of a person's health status (Long and Settle, 1984). Age reflects two opposing influences. On the one hand poorer health status creates a greater demand for health care services while on the other hand as a person grows older mobility limitations may impede access to health care services. Overall, it is hypothesized that age will be associated with an increase in the likelihood of having contact with a physician and with an increase in the number of physician visits.

2) The research on education and use of physician services is somewhat conflicting. A study by Stoller (1982) found that as years of education increases the likelihood of having contact with a physician increase but education had no effect on volume of services. This finding was supported by Branch and Nemeth (1985) who found that increasing years of education was associated with an increase in the likelihood of having contact with a physician. On the other hand, in Wolinsky and Johnson's (1991) analysis of data from the Longitudinal Study on Aging, education was associated with an increase in the number of physician visits among those with at least one visit, but had no effect on physician contact.

3) In an extensive review of the literature on gender and health care utilization Verbrugge (1985) reports that a number of investigators propose that women are more sensitive to illness symptoms than are men, that women are more likely to label these symptoms as physical illness, and that women are more likely than their male counterparts to seek medical care. Despite contradictory evidence regarding the linkage between gender and utilization, accounting for health status in an analysis (Krause, 1990), it is hypothesized that men will be less likely to report contact with a physician and will report fewer physician visits as compared with women.

4) There is some indication that household composition may be responsible for some of the variation in the use of physician services by the elderly. Elderly people living alone are significantly less likely to see a physician during the year as compared with their counterparts living with a relative (Long and Settle, 1984). Moreover, the level of physician use by those living alone is significantly less than for those living with a relative. Some conjectures for this include: elderly persons living alone may encounter greater transportation difficulties than those persons living with a relative, or other household members may be more likely to care-seeking.

5) The effect of race on access to and utilization of medical care services is presumed to be diminished by a variety of forces such as: Medicare; the growth of social programs such as Medicaid; and changes in racial attitudes (Long and Settle, 1984). It is questionable whether race will have a direct effect on utilization, however, its role as a mediating variable will be evaluated. Race is expected to have an indirect effects on use via perceived access and attitude but the direction is not clear.

Enabling Characteristics

6) Prior to Medicare the higher income elderly used more health services than the lower income elderly. Since the inception of the Medicare program income has decreased in importance in explaining variation of medical care use among elderly people. While income is not expected to influence utilization directly it is expected to influence use indirectly via concern with the cost

of care. Low income elderly who do not have Medicaid or private insurance supplementing Medicare may be more concerned with the cost of care because of copayments and deductibles, resulting in lower utilization but having no effect on the likelihood of having at least one contact with a physician.

7) Availability of Medicaid as an additional source of insurance has been found to increase the number of physician visits (Evash-wick et al., 1984; Wolinsky and Coe, 1984). In addition elderly people who had private insurance in addition to Medicare had an increase in the number of reported physician visits (Wolinsky and Coe, 1984; Eve, 1988). This relationship was noted to hold for white elderly but not for black elderly (Keith and Jones, 1990).

8) Having a regular source of care has been found to be positively associated with physician visits among elderly people living in the community (Wright, Creecy and Berg, 1979; Branch et al., 1981; Wolinsky et al., 1983). In addition, characteristics of the usual source of care (for example, private, emergency depart-ment, clinic) have also been associated with physician contact and volume of services (Stoller, 1982).

9) Elderly people living in urban areas are only slightly more likely to have contact with a physician during a year's time; however, among users of care, urban elders receive 21 percent more care than rural dwellers (Long and Settle, 1984).

10) The availability of social support has been positively associated with physician visits (Coulton and Frost, 1982; Arling, 1985).

Need-for-Care Characteristics

11, 12 and 13) Need-for-care has consistently been shown to be the primary factor in determining use of health care among older adults (see discussion in Chapter II).

REFERENCES

Aday, L., & Andersen, R. (1975). *Access to Medical Care.* Ann Arbor: Health Administration Press.

Aday, L. A., & Andersen, R. (1974). A framework for the study of access to medical care. *Health Services Research, 9*:208-220.

American Medical Association: Council on Ethical and Judicial Affairs (1990). Coucil Report: Black-White Disparities in Health Care. *Journal of the American Medical Association, 263*:2344-2346.

Alonzo, A. A. (1986). The impact of the family and lay others on care-seeking during life-threatening epidsodes of suspected coronary artery disease. *Social Science and Medicine, 22*:1297-1311.

Andersen, R. (1968). *Behavioral Model of Families' Use of Health Services* No. Research Series no. 25). Chicago, IL: Center for Health Administration Studies, University of Chicago.

Andersen, R., & Aday, L. A. (1978). Access to medical care in the U.S.: Realized and potential. *Medical Care, 16*:533-546.

Andersen, R., & Newman, J. F. (1973). Societal and individual determinants of medical care utilization in the United States. *Milbank Memorial Fund Quarterly, 51*:95-124.

Anderson, J. G. (1973). Health Services Utilization: Framework and Review. *Health Services Research, 8*:184-199.

Arber, S., & Ginn, J. (1993). Gender and inequalities in health in later life. *Social Science and Medicine, 36*:33-46.

Arling, G. (1985). Interaction effects in a multivariate model of physician visits by older people. *Medical Care, 23*:361-371.

Bausell, R. B. (1986). Health seeking behavior among the elderly. *The Gerontologist, 26*:556-569.

Becker, L. B., Han, B. H., Meyer, P. M., Wright, F. A., Rhodes, K. V., Smith, D. W., & Barrett, J. (1993). Racial differences in the incidence of cardiac arrest and subsequent survival. *New England Journal of Medicine, 329*:600-606.

Becker, M. H., & Maiman, L. A. (1983). Models of Health-Related Behavior. In D. Mechanic (Eds.), *Handbook of Health, Health Care and the Health Professions* (pp. 539-568). New York: Free Press.

Berkanovic, E., & Telesky, C. (1982). Social networks, beliefs, and the decision to seek medical care: An analysis of congruent and incongruent patterns. *Medical Care, 20*:1018-1026.

Berkanovic, E., Telesky, C., & Reeder, S. (1981). Structural and social psychological factors in the decision to seek medical care for symptoms. *Medical Care, 19*:693-709.

Berki, S. E., & Ashcraft, M. L. (1979). On the analysis of ambulatory utilization: An investigation of the roles of need, access and price as predictors of illness and preventive visits. *Medical Care, 17*:1163-1181.

Bernard, H. R., Killworth, P., Kronefeld, D., & Sailer, L. (1984). The problem of informant accuracy: The validity of retrospective data. *Annual Review of Anthropology, 13*:495-517.

Bice, T. W., Eichhorn, R. L., & Fox, P. D. (1972). Socioeconomic status and use of physician visits: A reconsideration. *Medical Care, 10*:261-271.

Blustein, J. & Weitzman, B.C. (1995). Access to Hospitals with High-Technology Cardiac Services: How is Race Important? *American Journal of Public Health, 85*:345-351.

Bollen, K.A. (1989) *Structural Equations With Latent Variables.* New York: Wiley.

Branch, L., Jette, A., Evashwick, C., Polansky, M., Rowe, G., & Diehr, P. (1981). Toward understanding elders' health service utilization. *Journal of Community Health, 7*:80-92.

Branch, L. G., & Nemeth, K. T. (1985). When elders fail to visit physicians. *Medical Care, 23*:1265-1275.

Brody, E. M., Kleban, M., H., & Moles, E. (1983). What older people do about their day-to-day mental and physical health symptoms. *Journal of the American Geriatrics Society, 31*:489-498.

Burns, R. B., Moskowitz, M. A., Ash, A., Kane, R. L., Finch, M. D., & Bak, S. M. (1992). Self-report versus medical record functional status. *Medical Care, 30*:MS85-MS95.

Chatters, L. M., Taylor, R. J., & Jackson, J. S. (1986). Size and composition of the informal helper networks of elderly blacks. *Journal of Gerontology, 40*:605-614.

Cleary, P., & Jette, A. (1984). The validity of self-reported physician utilization measures. *Medical Care, 22*:796-803.

Cleary, P. D., & Angel, R. (1984). The analysis of relationships involving dichotomous dependent variables. *Journal of Health and Social Behavior*, *25*:334-348.

Coe, R. M., Wolinsky, F. D., Miller, D. K., & Prendergast, J. M. (1984). Social network relationships and use of physician services. *Research on Aging*, *6*:243-256.

Cooper, R.S., Simmons, B. & Castaner A. (1986). Survival Rates and Prehospital Delay During Myocardial Infarction Among Black Persons. *American Journal of Cardiology*, 57:208-211.

Cornoni-Huntley, J., Blazer, D. G., Lafferty, M. E., Everett, D. F., Brock, D. B., & Farmer, M. E. (1990). *Established Populations for Epidemiologic Studies of the Elderly: Resource Data Book Volume II* (NIH Publication No. 90-495). National Institute on Aging. U.S. Department of Health and Human Services. Public Health Service. National Institutes of Health.

Cornoni-Huntley, J., Brock, D. B., Ostfeld, A. M., Taylor, J. O., & Wallace, R. B. (1986). *Established Populations for Epidemiologic Studies of the Elderly: Resource Data Book* (NIH Publication No.86-2443). National Institute on Aging. Department of Health and Human Services. Public Health Service. National Institutes of Health.

Coulton, C., & Frost, A. K. (1982). Use of social and health services by the elderly. *Journal of Health and Social Behavior*, *23*:330-339.

Counte, M. A., & Glandon, G. L. (1990). Health beliefs, attitudes, and behavior of older persons: An analysis of advances in research and future directions. In S. M. Stahl (Eds.), *The Legacy of Longevity: Health and Health Care in Later Life* (pp. 165-185). Newbury Park: Sage.

Counte, M. A., & Glandon, G. L. (1991). A panel study of life stress, social support, and the health services utilization of older persons. *Medical Care*, *29*:348-361.

Crawford, S. L., McGraw, S. A., Smith, K. W., McKinlay, J. B., & Pierson, J. E. (1994). Do blacks and whites differ in their use of health care for symptoms of coronary heart disease? *American Journal of Public Health*, *84*:957-964.

Davis, K. (1975). Equal treatment and unequal benefits: the medicare program. *Milbank Memorial Fund Quarterly*, *53*:449-472.

Davis, K., Lillie-Blanton, M., Lyons, B., Mullan, F., Powe, N., & Rowland, D. (1987). Health care for black Americans: The public sector role. *Milbank Quarterly, 65*:213-247.

Donabedian, A. (1973). *Aspects of Medical Care Administration: Specifying Requirements for Health Care.* Commonwealth Fund: Harvard University Press.

Ell, K., Haywood, L.J., sobel, E., deGuzman, M., Blumfield, D, & Ning, J.P. (1994). Acute Chest Pain in African Americans: Factors in the Delay in Seeking Emergency Care. *American Journal of Public Health, 84*:965-970.

Escarce, J. J., Epstein, K. R., Colby, D. C., & Schwartz, J. S. (1993). Racial differences in the elderly's use of medical procedures and diagnostic tests. *American Journal of Public Health, 83*:948-954.

Evashwick, C., Rowe, G., Diehr, P., & Branch, L. (1984). Factors explaining the use of health care services by the elderly. *Health Services Research, 19*:357-382.

Eve, S. B. (1988). A longitudinal study of use of health care services among older women. *Journal of Gerontology: Medical Sciences, 43*:M31-39.

Farmer, F. (1993). A literature review of health issues of the rural elderly. *The Journal of Rural Health, 9*:68-72.

Ferraro, K. F. (1980). Self-ratings of health among the old and the old-old. *Journal of Health and Social Behavior, 21*:377-383.

Fillenbaum, G. G., Hanlon, J. T., Corder, E. H., Ziqubu-Page, T., Wall, W. E., & Brock, D. (1993). Prescription and nonprescription drug use among black and white community-residing elderly. *American Journal of Public Health, 83*:1577-1582.

Fitti, J. E., & Kovar, M. G. (1987). The Supplement on Aging to the 1984 National Health Interview Study. In Vital and Health Statistics, Ser.1, No.21. (DHHS Pub. No. (PHS)). Washington, DC: U.S. Government Printing Office.

Fries, J. F. (1990). The compression of morbidity: Near or far? *Milbank Quarterly, 67*:209-231.

Garrett, J. M. (1993). Overview of Biostatistics. Cecil G. Sheps Center for Health Services Research: University of North Carolina at Chapel Hill.

Garrett, J. M., Harris, R. P., Norburn, J. K., Patrick, D. L., & Danis, M. (1993). Life-sustaining treatments during terminal illness: Who wants what? *Journal of General Internal Medicine, 8*:361-368.

Gatsonis, C.A., Epstein, A.M., Newhouse, J.P., Normand, S.L., & McNeil, B.J. (1995). Variations in the Utilization of an Acute Myocardial Infarction: An Analysis Using Hierarchical Logistic Regression. *Medical Care, 33*:625-642.

Getzen, T. E. (1991). Population Aging and the Growth of Health Expenditures. Presented at the Association for Health Services Research 10th Annual Meeting. San Diego, CA:

Gibson, R. C., & Jackson, J. S. (1992). The black oldest old: Health, functioning, and informal support. In R. M. Suzman, D. P. Willis, & K. G. Manton (Eds.), *The Oldest Old* Oxford: Oxford University Press.

Glandon, G. L., Counte, M. A., & Tancredi, D. (1992). An analysis of physician utilization by elderly persons: Systematic differences between self-report and archival information. *Journal of Gerontology: Social Sciences, 47*:S245-S252.

Goldsteen, R.L., Counte, M.A. & Goldsteen. (1994). Examining the Relationship Between Health Locus of Control and the Use of Medical Care Services. *Journal of Aging and Health, 6*:314-335.

Gujarati, D. N. (1988). *Basic Econometrics* (2nd Ed.). New York: McGraw-Hill.

Haug, M. R. (1981). Age and medical care utilization patterns. *Journal of Gerontology, 36*:103-111.

Health Care Financing Administration. (1992). *Monitoring Utilization of and Access to Services for Medicare Beneficiaries Under Physician Payment Reform. Report to Congress, FY 1992*. Health Care Financing Administration. Baltimore, MD.

Health Care Financing Administration. (1993). *Monitoring Utilization of and Access to Services for Medicare Beneficiaries Under Physician Payment Reform. Report to Congress, FY 1993*. Health Care Financing Administration. Baltimore, MD.

Health Care Financing Administration. (1994). *Monitoring Utilization of and Access to Services for Medicare Beneficiaries Under Physician Payment Reform. Report to Congress, FY 1994*. Health Care Financing Administration. Baltimore, MD

Hershey, J. C., Luft, H. S., & Gianaris, J. M. (1975). Making sense out of utilization data. *Medical Care, 13*:838-854.

Herzog, A., & Rogers, W. (1988). Age and response rates to interview sample surveys. *Journal of Gerontology, 43*:200-205.

High-Cost Users of Medicare Services. (1995). *Health Care Financing Review*, Statistical Supplement:36-37

Hulka, B. S., & Wheat, J. R. (1985). Patterns of utilization: The Patient perspective. *Medical Care, 23*:438-460.

Institute of Medicine (US): Committee on Monitoring Access to Personal health Care Services. (1993) *Access to Health Care in America.* National Academy Press.

Jackson, M., Kolodny, B., & Wood, J. L. (1982). To be old and black: The case for double jeopardy on income and health. In R. C. Manuel (Eds.), *Minority Aging: Sociological and Social Psychological Issues* (pp. 77-82). Wesport, CT: Greenwood Press.

Javitt, J.J., McBean, & A.M., Nicholson, G.A. (1991). Undertreatment of Glaucoma Among Black Americans. *New England Journal of Medicine*, 325:1418-1422.

James, S.A. (1989). Coronary Heart Disease in Black Americans: Suggestions for research on Psychosocial Factors. *American Heart Journal*, 113:833-838.

Jette, A. M., Cummings, K. M., Brock, B. M., Phelps, M. C., & Naessens, J. (1981). The structure and reliability of health belief indices. *Health Services Research, 16*:81-98.

Kane, R. A., & Kane, R. L. (1980). *Assessing the Elderly: A Practical Guide to Measurement.* Lexington, MA: Lexington Books.

Kane, R. L., & Kane, R. A. (1990). Health care for older people: Organizational and policy issues. In R. H. Binstock & L. K. George (Eds.), *Handbook of Aging and the Social Sciences* (pp. 415-437). San Diego, CA: Academic Press.

Kasl, S. (1974). The Health belief model and behavior related to chronic illness. In M. Becker (Eds.), *The Health Belief Model and Personal Health Behavior* (pp. 106-127). Thorofare, NJ: Slack Press.

Katz, S., Downs, T. D., Cash, H. R., et al., (1970). Progress in the development of an index of ADL. *The Gerontologist, 10*:20-30.

Katz, S., Ford, A., Moskowitz, R., Jackson, B., & Jaffe, M. (1963). Studies of illness in the aged. The Index of ADL: A standardized measure of biological and psychosocial function. *Journal of the American Medical Association, 185*:914-919.

Keith, V. M., & Jones, W. (1990). Determinants of health services utilization among the black and white elderly. *Journal of Health and Social Behavior, 1*:73-87.

Kirscht, J. (1974). The health belief model and illness behavior. In M. Becker (Eds.), *The Health Belief Model and Personal Health Behavior* (pp. 128-143). Thorofare, NJ: Slack Press.

Kleinbaum, D. G., Kupper, L. L., & Muller, K. E. (1988). *Applied Regression Analysis and Other Multivariable Methods* (2nd Ed.). Boston: PWS-Kent.

Kmenta, J. (1986). *Elements of Econometrics* (2nd Ed.). New York: Macmillan.

Kovar, M. G. (1986). Expenditures for the medical care of elderly people living in the community in 1980. *Milbank Memorial Fund Quarterly, 64*:100-132.

Kovar, M. G., & Feinlieb, M. (1991). Older Americans present a double challenge: Preventing disability and providing care. *American Journal of Public Health, 81*:287-88.

Krause, N. (1990). Illness Behavior in Late Life. In R. H. Binstock & L. K. George (Eds.), *Handbook of Aging and the Social Sciences* (pp. 227-244). New York: Academic Press.

Krout, J. A. (1983a). Correlates of service utilization among the rural elderly. *The Gerontologist, 23*:500-504.

Krout, J. A. (1983b). Knowledge and use of services by the elderly: A critical review of the literature. *International Journal of Aging and Human Development, 17*:153-167.

Letsch, S. W., Lazenby, H. C., Levitt, K. R., & Cowan, C. A. (1993). National health expenditures, 1991. *Health Care Financing Review, 14*:1-17.

Leventhal, E., & Prohaska, T. (1986). Age, symptom interpretation and health behavior. *Journal of the American Geriatrics Society, 34*:185-192.

Liang, J. (1986). Self-reported physical health among aged adults. *Journal of Gerontology, 41*:248-260.

Link, C. R., Long, S. H., & Settle, R. F. (1980). Cost-sharing, supplementary insurance, and health services utilization among the Medicare elderly. *Health Care Financing Review*, *2*:25-31.

Link, C. R., Long, S. H., & Settle, R. F. (1982a). Access to medical care under Medicaid: Differentials by race. *Journal of Health Politics, Policy and Law*, *7*:345-65.

Link, C. R., Long, S. H., & Settle, R. F. (1982b). Equity and the utilization of health care services by the Medicare elderly. *Journal of Human Resources*, *17*:195-212.

Linn, B. S., & Linn, M. W. (1980). Objective and self-assessed health in the old and very old. *Social Science and Medicine*, *14*:311-315.

Long, S. H., & Settle, R. F. (1984). Medicare and the disadvantaged elderly: Objectives and outcomes. *Milbank Quarterly*, *62*:609-656.

Maddala, G. (1983). *Limited-Dependent and Qualitative Variables in Econometrics*. Cambridge: Cambridge University Press.

Magaziner, J. (1992). The use of proxy respondents in health studies of the aged. In R. B. Wallace & R. F. Woolson (Eds.), *The Epidemiologic Study of the Elderly* Oxford: Oxford University Press.

Manton, K. G., Patrick, C. H., & Johnson, K. W. (1987). Health differentials between blacks and whites: Recent trends in mortality and morbidity. *Milbank Quarterly*, *65*:129-199.

Manuel, R. C. (Ed.). (1982). *Minority Aging: Sociological and Psychological Issues*. Westport, CT: Greenwood Press.

Manuel, R. C., & Reid, J. (1982). A comparative demographic profile of the minority and nonminority aged. In R. C. Manuel (Eds.), *Minority Aging: Sociological and Social Psychological Issues* (pp. 31-52). Westport, CT: Greenwood Press.

Markides, K. S., & Mindel, C. H. (Eds.). (1987). *Aging and Ethnicity*. Newbury Park: Sage.

Mechanic, D. (1979). Correlates of physician utilization. *Journal of Health and Social Behavior*, *20*:387-96.

McBean, A.M., & Gornick, M. (1994). Differences by Race in the Rates of Procedures Performed in Hospitals for Medicare Beneficiaries. *Health Care Financing Review*, *15*:77-90.

Mickey, R. M., & Greenland, S. (1989). The impact of confounder selection criteria on effect estimation. *American Journal of Epidemiology*, *129*:125-137.

Mossey, J. M., Havens, B., & Wolinsky, F. D. (1989). The consistency of formal health care utilization. In M. Ory & K. Bond (Eds.), *Aging and Health Care: Social Science and Policy Perspectives* (pp. 81-99). New York: Routledge.

Mossey, J. M., & Shapiro, M. (1982). Self-rated health: A predictor of mortality among the elderly. *American Journal of Public Health*, *72*:800-808.

Mutran, E. (1985). Intergenerational family support among blacks and whites: Response to culture or to socioeconomic differences. *Journal of Gerontology: Social Sciences*, *40*:S382-S389.

Mutran, E., & Ferraro, K. F. (1988). Medical need and use of services among older men and women. *Journal of Gerontology: Social Sciences*, *43*:S162-S171.

National Center for Health Statistics,(1990). *Current Estimates from the National Health Interview Survey, 1989* (Vital and Health Statistics Series 10 No. No. 176).

Olshansky, S.J., Rudberg, M.A., Carnes, B.A., Cassel, C.K., & Brody, J.A. (1991). Trading off longer life for worsening health. *Journal of Aging and Health*, *3*:194-216.

Parks, A. G. (1988). *Black Elderly in Rural America: A Comprehensive Study*. Bristol, IN: Wyndham Hall Press.

Penchansky, R., & Thomas, J. W. (1981). The concept of access: Definition and relationship to consumer satisfaction. *Medical Care*, *19*:127-140.

Rice, T., & McCall, N. (1985). The extent of ownership and the characteristics of Medicare supplemental policies. *Inquiry*, *22*:188-200.

Ronis, D. L., & Harrison, K. A. (1988). Statistical interactions in studies of physician utilization: Promise and pitfalls. *Medical Care*, *26*:361-372.

Roos, N. P., & Shapiro, E. (1981). The Manitoba longitudinal study on aging: Preliminary findings on health care utilization by the elderly. *Medical Care*, *19*:644-657.

Rosenstock, I. (1974). Historical origins of the health belief model. In M. Becker (Ed.), *The Health Belief Model and Personal Health Behavior* (pp. 1-8). Thorofare, NJ: Slack Press.

Rosner, T. T., Namazi, K. H., & Wykle, M. L. (1988). Physician use among the old-old: Factors affecting variability. *Medical Care, 26*:982-991.

Rosow, I., & Breslau, N. (1966). A Guttman health scale for the aged. *Journal of Gerontology, 21*:556-559.

Russell, L. B. (1981). An aging population and the use of medical care. *Medical Care, 19*:633-643.

Safer, M. A., Tharps, Q. J., Jackson, T. C., & Leventhal, H. (1979). Determinants of three stages of delay in seeking care at a medical clinic. *Medical Care, 17*:11- 29.

Salber, E. J., Greene, S. B., Feldman, J. J., & Hunter, G. (1976). Access to health care in a Southern rural community. *Medical Care, 14*:971-986.

Schoenfeld, D. E., Malmrose, L. C., Blazer, D. G., Gold, D. T., & Seeman, T. E. (1994). Self-rated health and mortality in the high functioning elderly - a closer look at healthy individuals: MacArthur field study of successful aging. *Journal of Gerontology: Medical Sciences, 49*:M109-M115.

Seccombe, K. (1995). Health Insurance Coverage and Use of Services Among Low-Income Elders: Does Residence Influence the Relationship? *Journal of Rural Health, 11*:86-96.

Sechrest, L., & Hannah, M. (1990). The Critical importance of nonexperimental data. In L. Sechrest, E. Perrin, & J. Bunker (Eds.), *Research Methodology: Strengthening Causal Interpretations of Nonexperimental Data*, (pp. 1-8). U.S. Department of Health and Human Services. Public Health Service. Agency for Health Care Policy and Research.

Segall, A., & Chappell, N. L. (1989). Health care beliefs and the use of Medical and social services by the elderly. In S. J. Lewis (Ed.), *Aging and Health: Linking Research and Public Policy* (pp. 129-141). Chelsea, MI: Lewis Publishers.

Shapiro, E., & Roos, N. P. (1985). Elderly nonusers of health care services: Their characteristics and their health outcomes. *Medical Care, 23*:247-257.

Shapiro, M. F., Hayward, R. A., Freeman, H. E., Sudman, S., & Corey, C. R. (1989). Out-of-pocket payments and use of care for serious and minor symptoms: Results of a national survey. *Archives of Internal Medicine, 149*:1646-48.

Shapiro, M. F., Ware, J. E., & Sherbourne, C. D. (1986). Effects of cost sharing on seeking care for serious and minor symptoms: Results of a randomized controlled trial. *Annals of Internal Medicine, 104*:246-251.

Smyer, M. A. (1980). The differential usage of services by impaired elderly. *Journal of Gerontology, 35*:249-255.

Soldo, B. J., & Manton, K. G. (1985). Changes in the health status and service needs of the oldest old: Current patterns and future needs. *Milbank Memorial Fund Quarterly, 63*:286-323.

Spencer, D. E., & Berk, K. N. (1981). A limited information specification test. *Econometrica, 49*:1079-1085.

Stoller, E. P. (1982). Patterns of physician utilization by the elderly: A Multivariate Analysis. *Medical Care, 20*:1080-1089.

Stoller, E. P. (1993). Interpretation of symptoms by older people: A health diary study of illness behavior. *Journal of Aging and Health, 5*:58-67.

Stoller, E.P. & Forster, L.D. (1994). The Impact of Symptom Interpretation on Physician Utilization. *Journal of Aging and Health,* 6:507-534.

Strogatz, D. (1990). Use of Medical Care for Chest Pain: Differences Between Blacks and Whites. *American Journal of Public Health,* 80:290-294.

Taeuber, C. M. (1992). *Sixty-Five Plus in America* (Current Population Reports, Special Studies No. P23-178). U. S. Bureau of the Census. U.S. Government Printing Office, Washington, DC.

Tanner, J. L., Cockerham, W. C., & Spaeth, J. L. (1983). Predicting physician utilization. *Medical Care, 21*:360-369.

Taylor, R. J. (1985). The extended family as a source of support to elderly blacks. *The Gerontologist, 25*:488-495.

Udvarhelyi, I.S., Gatsonis, C., & Epstein, A.M. (1992). Acute Myocardial Infarction: Process of Care and Clinical Outcomes. *Journal of the American Medical Association,* 268:2530-2536.

162   *Racial Differences in Access to Health Care*

Ulbrich, P. M., & Bradsher, J. E. (1993). Perceived support, help seeking, and adaptation to stress among older black and white women living alone. *Journal of Aging and Health, 5*:365-386.

U.S. Department of Health and Human Service. (1991). *Aging in America: Trends and Projections.* No. DHHS Publication No.(FCoA)91-28001).

U.S. House of Representatives, Special Council on Aging (1994). Medicare and Medicaid's 25th Anniversary: Much Promised, Accomplished, and Left Unfinished. In P. R. Lee & C. L. Estes (Eds.), *The Nation's Health.* Boston: Jones and Bartlett.

Verbrugge, L. M. (1984). A health profile of older women with comparisons to older men. *Research on Aging, 6*:291-322.

Verbrugge, L. M. (1989). The twain meet: Empirical explanations of sex differences in health and mortality. *Journal of Health and Social Behavior, 30*:282-304.

Wan, T. T. (1982). Use of health services by the elderly in low-income communities. *Milbank Memorial Fund Quarterly, 60*:82-107.

Wan, T. T. H. (1989). The behavioral model of health care utilization by older people. In M. Ory & K. Bond (Eds.), *Aging and Health Care: Social Science and Policy Perspectives* (pp. 52-76). New York: Routledge.

Wan, T. T. H., & Soifer, S. J. (1974). Determinants of physician utilization: A causal analysis. *Journal of Health and Social Behavior, 15*:100-108.

Weissman, J. S., Stern, R., Fielding, S. L., & Epstein, A. M. (1991). Delayed access to health care: Risk factors, reasons, and consequences. *Annals of Internal Medicine, 114*:325-331.

Whittle, J., Conigliaro, J., Good, C. B., & Lofgren, R. P. (1993). Racial differences in the use of invasive cardiovascular procedures in the department of veterans affairs medical system. *New England Journal of Medicine, 329*:621-627.

Wolinsky, F. (1981). The problem for academic and entrepreneurial research in the use of health service: The case of unstable structural relationships. *Sociology Quarterly, 22*:207-213.

Wolinsky, F. D. (1990). *Health and Behavior Among Elderly Americans: An Age-Stratification Perspective.* New York: Springer Publishing.

Wolinsky, F. D., Aguirre, B. E., Fann, K.-J., Keith, V. M., Arnold, C. L., Niederhauer, J. C., & Dietrich, K. (1989). Ethnic differences in the demand for physician and hospital utilzation among older adults in major American cities: Conspicuous evidence of considerable inequalities. *Milbank Quarterly, 67*:412-449.

Wolinsky, F. D., Aguirre, B. E., Fann, L., Keith, V. M., Arnold, C. L., Niederhauser, J. C., & Dietrich, K. (1990). Ethnic differences in the demand for physician and hospital utilization among older adults in major American cities: Conspicuous evidence of considerable inequalities. *The Milbank Quarterly, 67*:412-449.

Wolinsky, F. D., Arnold, C. L., & Nallapati, I. V. (1988). Explaining the declining rate of physician utilization among the oldest-old. *Medical Care, 26*:544-553.

Wolinsky, F. D., & Coe, R. M. (1984). Physician and hospital utilization among noninstitutionalized elderly adults: An analysis of the Health Interview Survey. *Journal of Gerontology, 39*:334-341.

Wolinsky, F. D., Coe, R. M., Miller, D. K., Prendergast, J. M., Creel, M. J., & Chavez, M. N. (1983). Health services utilization among the nonistitutionalized elderly. *Journal of Health and Social Behavior, 24*:325-337.

Wolinsky, F. D., Coe, R. M., Mosely, R. R., & Homan, S. (1985). Veterans' and nonveterans' use of health services: A comparative analysis. *Medical Care, 23*:1358-1371.

Wolinsky, F. D., & Johnson, R. J. (1991). The use of health services by older adults. *Journal of Gerontology: Social Sciences, 46*:345-357.

Wolinsky, F. D., Mosely II, R. R., & Coe, R. M. (1986). A cohort analysis of the use of health services by elderly Americans. *Journal of Health and Social Behavior, 27*:209-219.

Wright, R., Creecy, R. F., & William, E. B. (1979). The black elderly and their use of health care services: A causal analysis. *Journal of Gerontological Social Work, 2*:11-28.

Yeatts, D. E., Crow, T., & Folts, E. (1992). Service use among low-income minority elderly: Strategies for overcoming barriers. *The Gerontologist, 32*:24-32.

Yelin, E. H., Kramer, J. S., & Epstein, W. V. (1983). Is health care use equivalent across social groups? A diagnosis-based study. *American Journal of Public Health, 73*:563-571.

Yergan, J., Flood, A. B., LoGerfo, J. P., & Diehr, P. (1987). Relationship between patient race and the intensity of hospital Services. *Medical Care, 25*, 592-603.

INDEX